Neurological Emergencies in Clinical Practice

T0188844

Abdul Qayyum Rana
John Anthony Morren

Neurological Emergencies in Clinical Practice

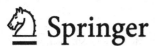 Springer

Abdul Qayyum Rana
MD, FRCPC, FRCP- Edin(Hon)
Parkinson's Clinic of Eastern
Toronto and Movement
Disorders Centre
Toronto
Canada

John Anthony Morren
MD/MBBS(Hons)
Neuromuscular Center
Neurological Institute
Cleveland Clinic
Ohio
USA

ISBN 978-1-4471-5190-6   ISBN 978-1-4471-5191-3   (eBook)
DOI 10.1007/978-1-4471-5191-3
Springer London Heidelberg New York Dordrecht

Library of Congress Control Number: 2013942486

I am very grateful to my teachers and colleagues, especially Dr. Arthur Walters, Dr. Pierre Bourque, and Dr. David Grimes, for their dedication to teaching which has served as an inspiration for me. I am also very thankful to Drs. Valerie Sim, Khurshid Khan, Syed Nizam, Lawrence Zumo, Ishtiaq Ahmad, Dar Dowlatshahi, and A.N. Rana, for their input and review of this manual. I am also thankful to Wasim Mansour, Asim Siddiqi, and Mohammad Abdullah Rana for their tireless support in completing this manual, and Evelyn Shifflett for drawing illustrations.

– Abdul Qayyum Rana

I am duly indebted to extraordinary teachers and mentors who supported my interest and pursuit of clinical and academic neurology: Dr. Surujpal Teelucksingh, Dr. Keith Aleong, and Dr. Azad Esack of the University of the West Indies, St. Augustine, Trinidad and Tobago; Dr. Efrain Salgado, Dr. Nestor Galvez-Jimenez, and Dr. Kerry Levin at Cleveland Clinic. Special thanks to Dr. Tarannum Khan for facilitating this particular joint venture with Dr. Rana. Deep gratitude goes out to my family for their enduring love and support throughout my long but rewarding years of education and training: my parents, Louis and Sumintra, and my motherly sisters Rena, Sharon, and Nesha. To my outstanding wife Divya who has been an exceptional source of help and encouragement. Finally, sincere thanks to our patients because of whom we are lifelong students.

– John Anthony Morren

Preface

This manual is designed to provide a stepwise approach for the management of neurological emergencies and is meant to primarily serve as a guide for medical students and residents on their neurology rotation. An attempt has been made to address day-to-day neurological issues in the emergency room, neurology ward/floor, and intensive care unit in an organized manner. Neurological problems are very complex but the protocols used in this book have been simplified so that trainees should not feel overwhelmed. This book is not to be taken as a comprehensive reference for neurology but more as a survival tool for those in training.

An attempt has been made to keep the format of the topics similar to help the trainee develop a stepwise approach to clinical problems. A brief introduction is provided for each topic, which is then divided into three main sections: stabilize the patient, identify the underlying cause, and treat the underlying cause. At the end, the discussion paragraphs provide some supplementary information not discussed under the previous headings. Some components of the initial history, physical examination, and investigations have been duly incorporated in the "stabilize the patient" section.

Most of the information presented in this book is considered generally accepted practice; however, the author and publisher are not responsible for any errors, omissions, or consequences from the application of this information and make no expressed or implied warranty of the contents of this publication. The reader is advised to check the package insert of each drug for its indication, dosage, and warnings. Suggestions to improve this publication are welcome and should be directed to the authors.

Toronto, ON, Canada   Abdul Qayyum Rana, MD, FRCPC,
                           FRCP-Edin (HON)
Cleveland, OH, USA   John Anthony Morren, MD/MBBS
                           (Hons)

Contents

Chapter 1
Coma

1. *Lethargy* is characterized by a state of drowsiness from which the patient can be aroused but cannot maintain that state of arousal and therefore relapses into drowsiness.
2. *Stupor* is characterized by incomplete arousal to painful/vigorous and continuous stimuli with absent or only minimal response to verbal command.
3. *Coma* is characterized by the total absence of awareness of self and relationship to the environment without any localizing or discrete defensive responses to external painful stimuli [1].

Stabilize the Patient

ABCs

1. Check the airway; if obstructed, clear by suction. Comatose patients are at risk of hypoxia and aspiration and need to be intubated to protect the airway and ensure adequate oxygenation. If there is any indication of respiratory depression in a lethargic or stuporous patient (especially if Glasgow Coma Scale is less than or equal to eight) or if the patient is comatose and has not been intubated already, proceed to intubation (using rapid induction) immediately. *If there is a potential cervical spine injury, the head should not be moved until radiographic assessment is done.* If there is a suspicion of cervical spine injury,

A.Q. Rana, J.A. Morren, *Neurological Emergencies in Clinical Practice*, DOI 10.1007/978-1-4471-5191-3_1,
© Springer-Verlag London 2013

the intubation should be done with in-line stabilization without extension of the neck or by surgical airway if necessary.
2. Check the vital signs and assess if the patient is hemodynamically stable. Place the patient on a cardiac monitor and pulse oximeter. Maintain the circulation; monitor the blood pressure, pulse, heart rate and rhythm continuously.

Focused History

Enquire about presenting symptoms and the onset from the available resources, including family members and paramedics, and review the emergency medical services sheet.

Focused Exam

1. Inspect the whole body for signs of trauma.
2. Do a focused neurological examination (see Glasgow Coma Scale (GCS) - Table 1.1) including observation of breathing pattern, pupil size and response, any eye deviation, facial symmetry (observe grimace), lateralization of movements in response to painful stimuli, posturing, deep tendon reflexes, and plantar responses (see section "Identify the Underlying Cause" for more detailed examination).
3. Perform cardiac and pulmonary auscultation.

STAT Labs and Treatments

1. Obtain finger-stick glucose. *Always give 100 mg of intravenous thiamine* before giving glucose 50 ml of D50W I.V., to prevent Wernicke's encephalopathy.
2. Get an ECG; start an I.V. line; draw STAT serum chemistry for electrolytes, glucose, BUN, creatinine, calcium, magnesium, AST, ALT, TSH, serum cortisol, PT/INR,

TABLE 1.1 Glasgow Coma Scale (GCS)

Eye opening	
Spontaneous	4
To voice	3
To pain	2
None	1
Best motor response	
Obeys commands	6
Localizes pain	5
Withdraws to pain	4
Flexor posturing	3
Extensor posturing	2
No response	1
Best verbal response	
Conversant and oriented	5
Conversant and disoriented	4
Inappropriate words	3
Incomprehensible sounds	2
No verbal response	1
Total score	3–15

CRP, ESR, serum osmolality, arterial blood gases, CBC, toxicology screen for opiates, barbiturates, cocaine, sedatives, antidepressants, and alcohol.

3. Start normal saline and insert a Foley catheter. Send urine for urine analysis with reflex culture and urine toxicology screen.

4. Obtain a STAT CT scan of the head to rule out intracranial causes such as epidural hematoma, subdural hematoma, intracerebral hemorrhage, subarachnoid hemorrhage, acute large ischemic stroke, other space-occupying lesion, herniation, midline shift, and other mass effects.

5. Obtain chest x-ray.
6. If the cause of coma is not clear, give naloxone 0.4–2 mg I.V. every 2–3 min PRN; you may need to give up to 10 mg to reverse coma caused by opiate intoxication. Flumazenil reverses the effects of benzodiazepines and is given at a dose of 0.2 mg I.V. over 30 s then 0.5 mg every 30 s up to total of 3 mg. Flumazenil should not be given if the patient had a seizure because it could precipitate seizures. *Caution as reversal effects for naloxone and flumazenil may be transient.*

Identify the Underlying Cause

Take Further History

Take a detailed history of onset, duration, circumstances, trauma, medications, recreational drug use, and past medical history.

Do Further Examination

For proper neurological assessment, turn off all administered sedation and allow time for effects to wear off.

1. Mental Status

   (a) Determine the patient's response to simple verbal commands such as "open your eyes" or "stick out your tongue" or "show me your right hand." Comprehension can be assessed by asking "yes" or "no" questions and asking patients their name; however, a comatose patient does not show any response to verbal commands or questions.

2. Cranial Nerve Examination

   (a) Examine the visual fields by response to visual threat stimuli. Some cortical functioning must be present if a response is observed. An asymmetry in response may

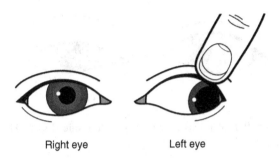

Right eye   Left eye

FIGURE I.I Left cranial nerve III palsy causing an ipsilateral dilated, fixed pupil; ptosis; and eye in down and out position

indicate a hemianopia or hemineglect/hemi-inattention.

(b) *Check fundi for papilledema. Papilledema results from prolonged elevation of intracranial pressure. Loss of spontaneous venous pulsations indicates probable increased intracranial pressure; however, in 15–20 % of normal population, the spontaneous venous pulsations are absent* [2].

(c) Examine pupils for size, shape, symmetry, and reactivity to light.

Round, regular, symmetric, and reactive to light: midbrain intact.

Unilateral dilated and fixed: uncal herniation or posterior communicating artery aneurysm due to cranial nerve III compression.

There may be ptosis and depression with external deviation of the ipsilateral eye as well (Fig. 1.1).

An acutely dilated unilateral fixed pupil requires urgent neurosurgical evaluation and intervention.

Bilateral dilated and fixed: hypoxic ischemic encephalopathy, opiate withdrawal, and intoxication with barbiturates, atropine, scopolamine, or glutethimide.

Pinpoint and reactive: pontine damage, opiate or cholinergic toxicity (e.g., pilocarpine). A magnifying lens may be used to determine the reactivity of pinpoint pupils to light.

Mid-position fixed or irregular: focal midbrain lesion.

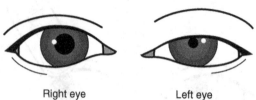

Right eye   Left eye

FIGURE I.2 Partial ptosis and miosis of left side due to Horner's syndrome

> *Unilateral small pupil or isolated miosis (especially with ipsilateral ptosis, facial anhidrosis, and enophthalmos)*: Horner's syndrome (Fig. 1.2); consider carotid or vertebral artery dissection [3].

(d) Observe the position of the eyes at rest.

> *Gaze deviation away from the side of hemiparesis*: hemispheric lesion contralateral to hemiparetic side.
>
> *Gaze deviation toward the side of hemiparesis ("wrong-way eyes")*: pontine lesion, hemispheric seizure focus contralateral to hemiparetic side, and thalamic lesion contralateral to hemiparetic side.
>
> *Downward gaze deviation*: lesions of the midbrain tectum. This may be accompanied by impaired pupillary reaction to light and convergence-retraction nystagmus called Parinaud's syndrome.
>
> *Ocular bobbing*: bilateral damage to the pontine horizontal gaze center. This consists of fast downward movements of both eyes with a slow return to primary position.

(e) Assess extraocular movements.

> *Oculocephalic (doll's eye) reflex: Check by actively turning the head side to side. Eyes should move conjugately in the direction opposite that of head turning.*
>
> *Oculovestibular reflex (cold caloric response): Prior to performing this, otoscopy is done to make sure that the patient has intact tympanic membranes. The head*

of the patient is tilted to 30° above the horizontal, and 50 cc of ice cold water is inserted into one ear canal with a butterfly tube. The normal response consists of tonic eye deviation toward the cold ear and a fast phase of nystagmus toward the opposite side (mnemonic: COWS = with Cold water, nystagmus corrective phase is Opposite and with Warm water, nystagmus corrective phase is on the Same side).

The absence of an oculovestibular response is indicative of deep coma.

Normally reactive pupils with an absent oculocephalic response or corneal reflex suggest a metabolic cause of coma.

(f) Test the corneal reflex by touching the cornea with a sterile gauze or cotton; always approach from the side and avoid inducing a visual threat response. The normal response results in reflex bilateral eye closure. The afferent limb of this reflex is mediated by cranial nerve V, and the efferent limb is mediated by cranial nerve VII.

(g) Facial asymmetry is assessed by looking at the grimace in response to painful stimuli or nasal tickle/nostril stimulation.

(h) Check the gag reflex by gently manipulating the endotracheal tube. Nurses monitoring intubated patients can also provide information on how much sedation was required to keep the patient from fighting the endotracheal tube.

(i) Check cough reflex with deep suctioning of the endotracheal tube.

(j) Check if the patient is breathing independently above the set ventilator respiratory rate.

3. Motor and Sensory Examination

(a) Observe the patient for any spontaneous movements. Preferential movements of one side of the body may be indicative of focal lesion, and myoclonus may suggest a metabolic cause of coma.

(b) Apply pressure with your fingers or knuckles to the sternum to determine if the patient has any localizing response.

> *Flexor response or decorticate posturing*: flexion and adduction of upper extremities and extension of the lower extremities resulting from damage to the corticospinal tract at or above the level of the upper midbrain (Fig. 1.3a).
>
> *Extensor response or decerebrate posturing*: extension and internal rotation of the upper extremities and extension of the lower extremities resulting from damage at or below the caudal midbrain-rostral pons level [1] (Fig. 1.3b).

(c) Apply pressure to the nail beds using the handle of reflex hammer on each extremity and observe for withdrawal response of limbs. Asymmetric response to painful stimuli also suggests a focal deficit.

(d) Assess the tone in the muscles of limbs for flaccidity or rigidity (including spasticity).

4. Deep Tendon Reflexes and Plantar Responses

(a) An asymmetry of deep tendon reflexes may indicate a focal deficit.

(b) An extensor plantar response (Babinski's sign) indicates a lateralizing upper motor neuron (corticospinal tract) lesion.

5. Meningeal Signs

> *Brudzinski's sign* is present if passive flexion of the patient's neck by the examiner results in flexion of the lower extremities.
>
> *Kernig's sign* is present if, with hip and knee in flexion, passive extension of the knee is restricted by hamstring spasm and/or pain. However, this may be difficult to check in a comatose patient.
>
> Meningeal signs have low sensitivity and specificity. Neck stiffness with extension and flexion but normal rotation is a more reliable sign of meningitis. *Also, meningismus is not specific to infection, but can be seen in subarachnoid hemorrhage as well.*

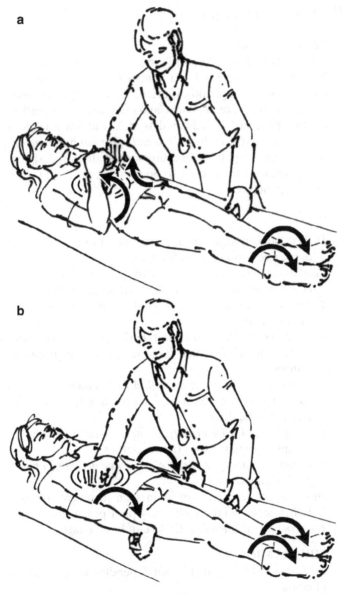

FIGURE 1.3 (a) Flexor or decorticate posturing: The arms are adducted and flexed at the elbow (often onto the chest), the wrists and fingers are flexed, and the lower extremities are extended. (b) Extensor or decerebrate posturing: adduction of the arms and extension and pronation of the forearms, together with extension of the lower extremities

Do Further Investigations

1. Lumbar Puncture
   If the patient has been febrile in last 24 h or complains of headaches, consider doing a lumbar puncture to rule out meningitis or encephalitis. If there is history of acute onset of extremely severe headache and the CT scan is negative, lumbar puncture is indicated to rule out subarachnoid hemorrhage. *Always do a CT scan before lumbar puncture* in a comatose patient because an infratentorial space-occupying lesion may cause brainstem herniation during a lumbar puncture.

2. EEG

   Diffuse background slowing: seen in almost all cases of depressed level of consciousness

   Continuous spike and wave activity in a stuporous or confused patient: nonconvulsive status epilepticus

   Triphasic waves: hepatic encephalopathy, renal and pulmonary failure

   PLEDS (periodic lateralizing epileptiform discharges): herpes encephalitis and large destructive hemispheric lesions

   Beta activity in combination with diffuse slowing: suggests overdose with barbiturates, benzodiazepines, or sedative hypnotic drugs

   Focal spike and wave activity: a single irritative focus as in complex partial (focal) onset seizures

   Generalized paroxysmal spike and wave activity: generalized seizures

   Burst suppression pattern: often seen in severe hypoxic-ischemic brain injury with very poor prognosis

   Electrocerebral silence: indicative of brain death

3. MRI and MRA
   MRI and MRA may be needed depending upon the cause of coma.

Causes of Coma

The coma may be due to structural, infectious, seizure-related, toxic, metabolic, systemic, and psychogenic causes. The structural causes are responsible for approximately a third of cases.

1. Structural Causes
   (a) Trauma: epidural hematoma, subdural hematoma, traumatic intracerebral and subarachnoid hemorrhage, concussion, and diffuse axonal injury
   (b) Vascular: cerebellar, brainstem, intracerebral, or subarachnoid hemorrhage; large hemispheric infarction with midline shift and mass effect or brainstem infarction; venous sinus thrombosis; hypertensive encephalopathy; vasculitis
   (c) Neoplasm: primary or metastatic neoplasm or non-metastatic complications of malignancy or immunosupression such as progressive multifocal leukoencephalopathy (PML)
2. Infections: meningitis, encephalitis, and brain abscess.
3. Seizure: status epilepticus or postictal state.
4. Toxic: drug intoxication or withdrawal (opiates, barbiturates, cocaine, alcohol) and heavy metals.
5. Metabolic: acid–base disturbances; hypo- or hyperglycemia; electrolyte disturbances like hypo- or hypercalcemia and hypo- or hypernatremia; liver, kidney, adrenal, and thyroid disorders; and thiamine deficiency.
6. Systemic: hypoxic ischemic encephalopathy secondary to cardiac and pulmonary causes, carbon monoxide poisoning, and hypo- or hyperthermia.
7. Psychogenic: These are infrequently encountered by neurologists but can be suspected with normal neurological examination and dramatic response to cold water caloric testing.

Treat the Underlying Cause

Treatment depends on the underlying cause of coma.

1. Raised intracranial pressure is often seen in structural causes of coma.

    (a) Elevate the head of the patient.
    (b) Intubate using rapid induction to minimize transient elevation in blood pressure.
    (c) Hyperventilate to lower $paCO_2$ to 25–30 mmHg and induce intracerebral vasoconstriction which helps reduce intracerebral pressure [4].
    (d) Neurosurgical consultation is required.

2. Cytotoxic edema, as seen in stroke, can cause herniation.

    (a) Start the patient on 20 % mannitol 1 g/kg with rapid I.V. infusion. Titrate to a serum osmolality of 300–320. This only has a temporary effect but is helpful when the patient is waiting for the neurosurgical intervention.
    (b) Neurosurgical consultation is required.

3. Vasogenic edema, as seen in brain tumors and abscesses, is treated with dexamethasone I.V. 10 mg bolus followed by 4 mg every 6 h with G.I. prophylaxis (gastric mucosal protection) and blood glucose monitoring.

4. If meningitis or encephalitis is suspected, treatment is started immediately (see Chap. 9), without delay pending the arrangements for lumbar puncture.

    (a) Meningitis: ceftriaxone 2 g I.V. every 12 h.
    (b) If *Listeria* is suspected, add ampicillin 1–2 g I.V. every 3–4 h.
    (c) If *Staphylococcus* is suspected, add vancomycin 1 g I.V. every 12 h. (In Ontario, Canada, vancomycin is also used for *Streptococcus pneumoniae* coverage as the resistance rate in Ontario is over 20 %).
    (d) Use de*xamethasone which may decrease morbidity and mortality: with or shortly (10–20 min) before the first dose of antibiotic in all non-immunosuppressed and previously well adults with (suspected or confirmed) pneumococcal meningitis at a dose of 10 mg every 6 h for 4 days and children at a dose of 0.15 mg/kg every*

6 h for 4 days for (suspected or confirmed) Haemophilus influenzae type b and pneumococcal meningitis [5].

(e) If herpes encephalitis is suspected, add acyclovir 10 mg/kg I.V. every 8 h.

5. Toxic and metabolic causes are treated accordingly.

Discussion

Prognosis of Coma

The prognosis of coma depends primarily upon the cause of coma. Usually coma from metabolic causes and drug intoxication has the most favorable prognosis followed by coma secondary to trauma, whereas coma from hypoxic ischemic encephalopathy carries the least favorable prognosis.

References

1. Posner JB, Saper CB, Schiff N, Plum F. Plum and Posner's diagnosis of stupor and coma. 4th ed. New York: Oxford University Press; 2007.
2. Agarwal S, Agarwal A, Apple DJ. Textbook of ophthalmology, vol. 1. New Delhi: Jaypee Brothers Medical Publishers; 2002.
3. Lee JH, Lee HK, Lee DH, Choi CG, Kim SJ, Suh DC. Neuroimaging strategies for three types of Horner syndrome with emphasis on anatomic location. AJR Am J Roentgenol. 2007;188(1):W74–81.
4. Milaković B, Dimitrijević I, Malenković V, Marković D, Pantić-Palibrk V, Gvozdenović L. Preoperative assessment and preparation of patients with diseases affecting the central nervous system. Acta Chir Iugosl. 2011;58(2):83–90.
5. Chaudhuri A, Martinez-Martin P, Kennedy PG, Andrew Seaton R, Portegies P, Bojar M, Steiner I, EFNS Task Force. EFNS guideline on the management of community-acquired bacterial meningitis: report of an EFNS Task Force on acute bacterial meningitis in older children and adults. Eur J Neurol. 2008;15(7):649–59.

Chapter 2
Delirium

Delirium or acute confusional state is characterized by a fluctuating level of consciousness with impairment of attention, perception, and thinking. Patients in a delirious state are usually agitated and may have hallucinations. Four primary features include disturbance of consciousness, disturbance of cognition, limited course, and external causation [1].

Stabilize the Patient

ABCs

1. Use a quiet room if possible. Provide reorientation and reassurance to the patient. If the patient is agitated, physical restraints should be avoided as much as possible but may be required to protect against injury, especially if the patient is pulling out I.V. lines.
2. Assess the airway and breathing rate and pattern, and look for signs of respiratory distress.
3. Check the vital signs and assess if the patient is hemodynamically stable. Provide I.V. fluids if needed. Place the patient on a cardiac monitor, pulse oximeter, and oxygen if required.

A.Q. Rana, J.A. Morren, *Neurological Emergencies in Clinical Practice,* DOI 10.1007/978-1-4471-5191-3_2, © Springer-Verlag London 2013

Focused History

Enquire about presenting symptoms and onset from the available resources. Ask if the change in mental state is acute or chronic (symptoms of delirium usually develop over 2–3 days).

Initial Labs and Treatments

1. Obtain finger-stick glucose. *Always give 100 mg of intravenous thiamine before giving glucose 50 ml of D50W I.V.,* to prevent Wernicke's encephalopathy.
2. Draw labs including basic chemistry, CBC with differential, ESR, CRP, ANA, RF, cardiac enzymes, electrolytes, glucose, AST, ALT, UA, calcium, magnesium, phosphorous, urine and serum toxicology, and alcohol level.
3. If fever is present, do urine and blood cultures and sensitivities.
4. Order blood gases, ECG, and chest x-ray.
5. Give I.V. normal saline if needed.

Identify the Underlying Cause

Take Further History

1. Ask family members if the patient has any history of underlying dementia, psychiatric condition, insomnia, alcohol or drug abuse, or a history of seizures or head injury.
2. Ask about any new medications started recently such as sedatives/hypnotics like benzodiazepines and opiates/opioids, trihexyphenidyl, benztropine, dopamine agonists such as pramipexole and ropinirole or levodopa, oxybutynin, digoxin, steroids, anticonvulsants, antiarrhythmics, antipsychotics, H2 blockers, and lithium.
3. Ask if there is any history of diabetes; hypertension; thyroid disease; psychiatric illness; renal, liver, pulmonary, or

cardiac condition; primary cancer, metastasis, or paraneo-plastic condition; or HIV.

4. Ask about the symptoms of pneumonia such as fever, cough, chest pain, or shortness of breath, or symptoms of urinary tract infection such as increased frequency of uri-nation, dysuria, and hematuria.

Do Further Examination

If the patient is agitated and interferes with assessment and investigations, then haloperidol 2–10 mg I.M. can be given, except in suspected alcohol withdrawal. Lorazepam 1–2 mg should be used in these patients.

1. Mental Status

   (a) Assess mental status and look for evidence of aphasia.
   (b) Check comprehension by responses to simple verbal commands.
   (c) Note speech and thought content.

2. Cranial Nerve Examination

   (a) Check the fundus for papilledema.
   (b) Check pupils for size, shape, regularity, and reactivity to light.

      Very small pupils: consider possible opiate intoxi-cation.
      Very enlarged pupils: consider anticholinergic intoxi-cation.

3. Motor and Sensory Examination

   (a) With a cooperative patient, check for pronator drift and rapid arm rolling (rapid alternating movements).
   (b) With a noncooperative patient, look for any asymme-try of spontaneous movements on both sides.
   (c) Response to noxious stimuli can be used if the patient cannot obey any commands.

(d) Assess the tone in the muscles of limbs for flaccidity or rigidity (including spasticity).

4. Deep Tendon Reflexes and Plantar Responses
5. Coordination

(a) Assess finger-nose-finger and heel-knee-shin tests if possible.
(b) Check gait for ataxia and instability with tandem and stress maneuvers.

6. Meningeal Signs

Brudzinski's sign is present if passive flexion of the patient's neck by the examiner results in flexion of the lower extremities.

Kernig's sign is present if, with hip and knee in flexion, passive extension of the knee is restricted by hamstring spasm and/or pain.

Meningeal signs have low sensitivity and specificity. Neck stiffness with extension and flexion but normal rotation is a more reliable sign of meningitis. Also, meningismus is not specific to infection, but can be seen in subarachnoid hemorrhage.

7. General Examination

Auscultate lungs and heart. *Inspect skin for herpetic rashes, erythema chronicum migrans, non-blanching petechial or purpuric rashes, livedo reticularis, etc.*

Do Further Investigations

If the patient is febrile or has a headache, focal deficit, any meningeal sign, or papilledema, further investigations are indicated.

1. CT Scan of the Head
2. Lumbar Puncture

If meningitis or encephalitis is suspected and the CT scan is negative for any focal lesions, lumbar puncture and CSF analysis are required.

Bacterial meningitis: polymorphonuclear pleocytosis, decreased glucose, and increased protein

Viral meningitis: lymphocytic pleocytosis, normal glucose, and increased protein

Encephalitis: (especially in herpetic cases) increased red cells and/or xanthochromia, lymphocytic pleocytosis, and normal glucose

3. EEG

Diffuse background slowing: seen in almost all cases of depressed level of consciousness

Continuous spike and wave activity in a stuporous or confused patient: nonconvulsive status epilepticus

Triphasic waves: hepatic encephalopathy and renal and pulmonary failure

PLEDS (periodic lateralizing epileptiform discharges): herpes encephalitis and large destructive hemispheric lesions

Beta activity in combination with diffuse slowing: suggests overdose with barbiturates, benzodiazepines, or sedative hypnotic drugs

Focal spike and wave activity: a single irritative focus as in partial (focal) onset seizures

Generalized paroxysmal spike and wave activity: generalized seizures

4. Brain MRI and MRA

MRI and MRA may be needed depending upon the cause of delirium.

Treat the Underlying Cause

Treatment depends on the underlying cause of delirium.

1. Medications

If the patient is on medications which seem to be responsible for delirium, these medications should be stopped.

2. Sepsis, Pneumonia, and Urinary Tract Infection

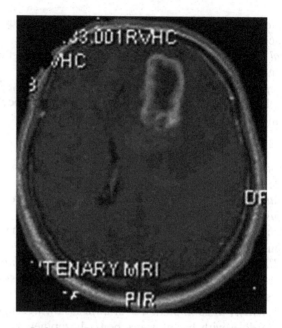

FIGURE 2.1 Left frontal ring-enhancing lesion on MRI characteristic of glioblastoma multiforme (Courtesy of Dr. J. Murphy)

Urinary tract infections in the elderly are the most common cause of delirium and must always be excluded.

If systemic causes such as sepsis, pneumonia, or UTI are found, treat with appropriate antibiotics, I.V. fluids, and blood pressure support.

3. Meningitis or Encephalitis

Please see Chap. 9 for details.

4. Focal Mass Lesions or Hemorrhage

Brain tumor, subdural or epidural hematoma, intracerebral hemorrhage, subarachnoid hemorrhage, and abscess usually can be seen on brain CT or MRI scan (Fig. 2.1), and treatment is given accordingly. *Neurosurgery consultation is required.*

In about 10 % of subarachnoid hemorrhage cases, the CT scan may not be diagnostic; therefore, a lumbar puncture for CSF analysis is required if subarachnoid hemorrhage is suspected.

5. Delirium Tremens

   Delirium tremens is usually seen more than 48 h after the last alcohol consumption. The patient may have fever, tachycardia, tachypnea, change in mental status, and hallucinations. The mortality is about 10–15 %. Treatment is as follows:

   (a) Thiamine 100 mg I.V. once daily to prevent acute worsening of Wernicke's encephalopathy and progression to Korsakoff's syndrome.
   (b) Chlordiazepoxide 25–50 mg every 6 h, titrated to symptoms or diazepam 5–10 mg I.V. load, then 2–5 mg I.V. every 30–60 min PRN.
   (c) Keep well hydrated with I.V. fluids.
   (d) Cardiac monitoring is required because arrhythmia can occur.
   (e) Tylenol® may be used PRN if no hepatic impairment is present.

6. Other Causes

   (a) *Hypoglycemia*: thiamine 100 mg I.V. followed by 50 ml of D50 water I.V. Internal medicine consultation is required.
   (b) *Hyperglycemia*: insulin drip and I.V. fluids. Correct acidosis, potassium, and other electrolyte abnormalities. Internal medicine consultation is required.
   (c) *Hyponatremia: Sodium must be corrected slowly, as too rapid a correction of hyponatremia may lead to central pontine or extra-pontine myelinolysis.* Internal medicine consultation is required.
   (d) *Uremia with renal failure*: hemodialysis. Internal medicine +/− nephrology consultation is required.
   (e) *Hypocalcaemia*: If severe, give 10 % calcium gluconate, 10–20 ml in 100 ml of D5W over half an hour.

Patients on digoxin need cardiac monitoring because calcium can potentiate digoxin toxicity. Internal medicine consultation is required.

(f) *Psychiatric causes*: Haloperidol 1–5 mg I.M. may be given initially. Psychiatry consultation is required.

(g) *Seizures*: Postictal confusion often follows a seizure. This improves over time. If there is a known history of seizures, then treatment should be directed toward preventing further seizures. (Please see Chap. 16 for details.)

(h) *Nonconvulsive status epilepticus*: If nonconvulsive status epilepticus is suspected, continuous EEG monitoring is required. Treat per protocol (see Chap. 16).

(i) *Demented patients*: Patients should be stabilized. A complete assessment of dementia should be done after the delirium resolves.

(j) *Parkinsonism*: Adjust antiparkinsonian medications and give I.V. fluids. Quetiapine 12.5–25 mg starting dose may be used.

(k) *Hepatic encephalopathy*: Patients may have a history of alcoholic cirrhosis, hepatitis, or carcinoma of the liver. Ammonia is increased and therefore dietary protein should be restricted. Lactulose 30–45 ml four times daily is given to induce diarrhea (increases stool acidity and sequesters bowel ammonia). Neomycin 2–4 g daily reduces the growth of ammonia-producing bacteria in the bowel. Diazepam 5–10 mg I.V. every 8 h is given. *Haloperidol should not be given*. Close monitoring with neurochecks should be instituted to detect early signs of increased intracranial pressure secondary to cerebral edema which may acutely develop.

(l) *Hypertensive encephalopathy*: This is a rare cause of delirium and occurs with markedly elevated blood pressure (systolic pressure usually above 220 mmHg and diastolic pressure above 120 mmHg). It is characterized by headache, confusion, irritability, and altered level of consciousness. Internal medicine consultation is required.

Discussion

Dementia

Demented patients may become delirious with a change in environment. This includes "sundowning" which often occurs in the hospital setting [2]. Active orientation strategies may be helpful in the prevention and management of sundowning and include having the patient in a room with an undraped window, making a large clock easily visible at all times, having familiar faces (including pictures) at bedside and frequent verbal reminders of current date, time, place, and persons.

History is very helpful to differentiate dementia from delirium. Dementia affects memory more than attention. Delirium may take days to weeks to clear, but the resolution is complete if there is no underlying dementia.

Prognosis

In frail elderly patients, delirium is associated with increased mortality [3]. Up to 40 % 1-year mortality has been reported after hospital discharge [4].

References

1. Deksnytė A, Aranauskas R, Budrys V, Kasiulevičius V, Sapoka V. Delirium: its historical evolution and current interpretation. Eur J Intern Med. 2012;23(6):483–6.
2. Balas MC, Rice M, Chaperon C, Smith H, Disbot M, Fuchs B. Management of delirium in critically ill older adults. Crit Care Nurse. 2012;32(4):15–26.
3. Siddiqi N, House AO, Holmes JD. Occurrence and outcome of delirium in medical in-patients: a systematic literature review. Age Ageing. 2006;35(4):350–64.
4. Wass S, Webster PJ, Nair BR. Delirium in the elderly: a review. Oman Med J. 2008;23(3):150–7.

Chapter 3
Dizziness and Vertigo

Dizziness is a very common complaint encountered in the neurology outpatient clinics as well as in the emergency departments. The term "dizzy" is often used nonspecifically, and it is essential to ascertain the precise nature of symptoms [1, 2].

Vertigo is considered a hallucination of movement (often that of spinning). If present, it more reliably implicates a neuro-otological etiology.

It is important to rule out potentially serious neurological conditions such as cerebellar hemorrhage or large cerebellar ischemic stroke which can lead to fatal complications such as herniation.

Stabilize the Patient

ABCs

1. Assess the airway and breathing rate, and look for signs of respiratory distress.
2. Check the vital signs and assess if the patient is hemodynamically stable. Check orthostatic vitals. A change in systolic BP within 3 min from supine to standing of at least 20 mmHg (or diastolic BP change of at least 10 mmHg) indicates orthostatic hypotension [3]. Provide I.V. fluids if needed, especially if orthostatic. Place the patient on a cardiac monitor, pulse oximeter, and oxygen if required.

A.Q. Rana, J.A. Morren, *Neurological Emergencies in Clinical Practice,* DOI 10.1007/978-1-4471-5191-3_3,
© Springer-Verlag London 2013

Focused History

Enquire about presenting symptoms and onset. *New-onset vertigo with alteration in level of consciousness is usually due to a potentially serious cause and is a neurological emergency.*

Focused Exam

Assess the mental status, cranial nerves, motor system including plantar responses, finger-nose-finger, heel-knee-shin test, and gait.

Initial Labs and Treatments

1. Obtain finger stick glucose.
2. Order an ECG.
3. Urine toxicology.

Identify the Underlying Cause

Take Further History

1. Ask the patient to describe the dizziness without using the word "dizziness". If they are not able to describe their symptoms clearly, try giving them four choices:

    (a) Spinning sensation or movement of self or environment, i.e., vertigo
    (b) Light-headedness or feeling of passing out, i.e., presyncope
    (c) Unsteadiness or feeling of imbalance
    (d) Floating sensation or like being on a boat

2. Take a detailed history of symptoms.

    (a) Are the symptoms episodic or continuous?
    (b) If episodic, how many episodes daily? How long does each episode lasts? Any triggers? Any relation to

head movement? Any relation to change in position such as standing up from a supine position? Any relation to straining/Valsalva?

(c)   Are symptoms more prominent in the morning, after meals, while urinating, or with hyperventilation?

3.   Ask about associated symptoms that might localize to the brainstem.

(a)   Visual impairment, double or blurred vision
(b)   Speech or swallowing problems
(c)   Weakness, numbness, tingling, or loss of sensation
(d)   Bowel or bladder problems
(e)   Tinnitus, hearing loss, sensation of fullness in the ears (which is usually due to inner ear pathology such as Ménière's disease)

4.   Ask if any new medications have been started recently.
5.   Ask if there is any history of psychiatric disorders.

Do Further Examination

1.   A complete neurological examination should be done. This includes testing mental status, cranial nerves, muscle bulk, tone, power, adventitious movements, deep tendon reflexes, plantar responses, station and coordination with gait and sensory assessment.
2.   Nystagmus should be checked in primary position as well as in all directions of gaze.

Peripheral causes of nystagmus: The nystagmus is usually rotational, may exhibit a latency of several seconds, and may extinguish with repetitive provocative maneuvers.

Central causes of nystagmus: The nystagmus is usually purely vertical, does not show any latency, does not extinguish with provocative maneuvers, and may have accompanying brainstem signs.

3.   The Barany or Dix-Hallpike maneuver should be performed (Fig. 3.1).

The patient is asked to sit with head turned to one side and neck hyperextended to 30°. Then the patient is made to lie down quickly, keeping the head in the same position relative to the body. This is repeated with the head turned to the opposite side. With a positive test, there is a latent period of 1–5 s followed by the acute onset of vertigo and rotatory nystagmus with the rapid component toward the affected side. Symptoms and visible nystagmus are typically 10–40 s in duration.

4. The Fukuda-Unterberger stepping test: The patient is blindfolded, extends both arms, and marches in place for 50 steps. A deviation/maximum rotation of more than 30° suggests asymmetrical labyrinthine function with the weaker side ipsilateral to the rotation.

5. Head thrust test: The patient's head is rotated 10–20° in the horizontal plane while focusing on the examiner's eyes directly forward. With unilateral vestibular weakness, there is a corrective saccade when rapid rotation occurs ipsilateral to the lesion. This test typically localizes to one or the other horizontal semicircular canal.

6. Examine the cardiovascular system. Assess for any correction in orthostatic vitals if the patient had I.V. fluid replacement. Check the pulse for regularity, auscultate heart sounds, and listen for carotid bruits.

7. Perform otoscopy to look for vesicles in the external ear canal (these are seen in Ramsay Hunt syndrome).

Do Further Investigations

1. CT Scan of the Head
   This should be obtained in new-onset vertigo especially if the patient is elderly or if there are any suggestions of a central cause. A head CT scan may also detect superior semicircular canal dehiscence which produces symptoms with straining.

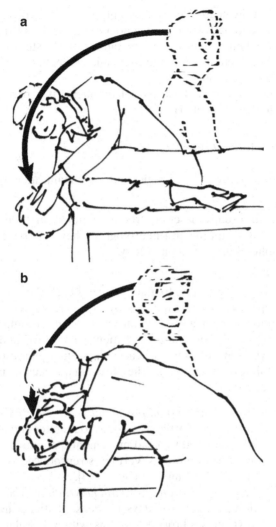

Figure 3.1 The Dix-Hallpike maneuver, a series of two steps: The patient sits on the table, facing forward, eyes open; the head is turned 45° to the left (a). The head is supported as the patient goes quickly from a sitting to supine position, ending with the head extended about 20°–30° off the edge of the table. The patient sustains this position for 30 s before returning to the upright position for another 30 s of observation. The maneuver is then repeated with the patient's head turned to the right (b). The test is considered positive if any of these maneuvers reproduce vertigo +/− nystagmus

2. MRI of the head, echocardiogram, Holter monitor, carotid ultrasound, and electronystagmography (ENG) as required. MRI is better than CT for visualizing the posterior fossa contents including the brainstem and cerebellum.

3. ENT Evaluation

   Depending upon the cause of dizziness (if a peripheral etiology is suspected)

Differential Diagnosis

Divide the approach to dizziness into two main categories:

1. Vertigo

   Patients usually describe "room spinning" or "self-spinning." If symptoms are neurological, they may be due to peripheral or central pathology.

   (a) *Peripheral Causes*

   These are related to inner ear pathology. The vertigo is episodic, may be induced by or worsened with head movement in any direction, and typically accompanied by nausea or vomiting. Patients may have auditory symptoms of tinnitus, hearing loss, aural pressure, and fullness in the ears. The three main causes are as follows:

   1. *Benign paroxysmal positional vertigo (BPPV)*: The duration of vertigo is seconds to minutes and is usually triggered by head movement. Patients have no auditory symptoms. Vertigo is reproduced by Dix-Hallpike testing (see Fig. 3.1) [4].

   2. *Vestibular neuronitis or viral labyrinthitis*: The duration of vertigo is days to weeks. Patients usually have no auditory symptoms with vestibular neuronitis but may have severe nausea and vomiting.

   3. *Ménière's disease*: The duration of vertigo is minutes to hours. Patients may have hearing loss, tinnitus, and aural pressure which they describe as fullness in the ear.

(b) *Central Causes*

Patients may give a history of weakness, numbness, dysphagia, dysarthria, visual problems, and bowel or bladder dysfunction. The duration is usually minutes to hours or is intractable. Causes include cerebellar or brainstem infarct, hemorrhage, tumor, abscess, head trauma, vertebrobasilar migraine, and multiple sclerosis, among others.

2. Non-vertigo

There are three main symptoms:

(a) *Light-Headedness, Feeling of Passing Out, or Presyncope*

The causes include postural hypotension, cardiac arrhythmias, aortic stenosis, dehydration, anemia, antihypertensive medications, and hypoglycemia. Patients might have profuse perspiration, palpitations, nausea, and generalized weakness. Symptoms usually occur when the patient is getting up from a supine position or after meals. Screen for orthostatic hypotension.

(b) *Unsteadiness or Disequilibrium*

This is the most common type of chronic dizziness. Medications such as sedatives and hypnotics may be responsible. The patient may have impaired vision, peripheral neuropathy, muscle weakness, arthritis, mechanical foot problems, or impaired joint position sense. Patients may complain of numbness, tingling, weakness, or incoordination of limbs which is worsened by walking and relieved by sitting or lying down. Screen for orthostatic hypotension in these patients as well. Further work-up with electrodiagnostic studies and orthopedics consultation may be required.

(c) *Floating Sensation*

This is usually associated with anxiety, stress, and other mood disorders. The patients may describe tingling sensations also. Associated symptoms include insomnia, fatigue, headache, and neck pain. The sensation can be exacerbated by hyperventilation or emotional stress.

Treat the Underlying Cause

Treat the underlying cause accordingly.

1. Benign Paroxysmal Positional Vertigo

    (a)   Advise bed rest and adequate fluid intake.

    (b)   Meclizine 12.5–25 mg three times daily or promethazine 12.5–25 mg three times daily may provide symptomatic benefit. Other treatments include benzodiazepines and ondansetron.

    (c)   Otolith repositioning exercises such as modified Epley's maneuver and vestibular rehabilitation with stationary eye and upper body movements, and gait and balance training may be helpful. Brandt and Daroff exercises are also effective in many cases.

Modified Epley's maneuver (Fig. 3.2) *consists of the following four important steps*:

1. The patient is asked to sit with head turned to the side of the "bad ear" determined by Dix-Hallpike testing. Then the patient quickly lies down, on his or her back, keeping the head turned and hyperextending the neck 45° over the end of the table.
2. While maintaining neck in hyperextension, the patient slowly turns the head to the good side.
3. Then the patient rolls over to the good side completely, with the head facing down toward the floor.
4. Finally, the patient slowly returns to a normal sitting position with the chin tilted down.

2. Ménière's Disease and a Superior Semicircular Canal Dehiscence Syndrome
   ENT consultation is required.
3. Vestibular Neuronitis/Viral Labyrinthitis
   Provide symptomatic treatment with antiemetics, adequate fluid intake, and bed rest.
4. Cardiac Causes
   ECG, Holter monitor, 2-D echocardiogram, and cardiology referral

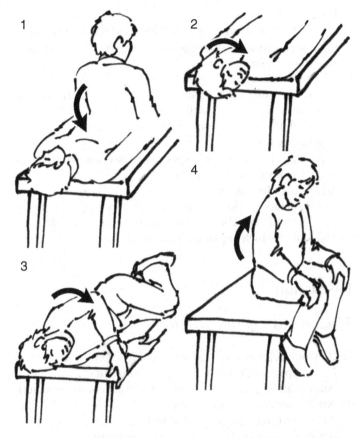

FIGURE 3.2 Modified Epley's maneuver, a canalith repositioning maneuver for benign positional vertigo.

Step 1. Lying down from sitting position with head extended 45° over the edge of table with impaired ear turned down 45°. This is maintained for 30 s.

Step 2. The head is rotated 90° in the opposite direction for another 30 s.

Step 3. The head and entire body is then further turned 90° (in the opposite direction) slowly, and the patient maintains this position for 30 s.

Step 4. The patient returns to the sitting position slowly with chin tilted down

5. Postural Hypotension

Treat the underlying cause. Advise good fluid intake, free salt intake, compression stockings, and slow rising from a seated or supine position.

6. TIA or Stroke

If TIA is suspected, brain MRI, Holter monitor, 2-D echocardiogram, lipid profile, and full stroke work-up are essential. Please see Chap. 18 for further details.

7. Psychiatric Causes

If psychiatric causes are suspected, reassurance and a psychiatric consultation are indicated.

8. Miscellaneous Causes

These include Parkinsonism, CNS tumors, CNS infections, head trauma, vertebrobasilar migraine, and multiple sclerosis, all of which are treated accordingly.

Discussion

Medications Causing Dizziness

1. Benzodiazepines, e.g., diazepam, chlordiazepoxide
2. Neuroleptic medications, e.g., phenothiazines
3. Antibiotics, e.g., gentamycin and streptomycin (ototoxicity)
4. Antihistamines, e.g., ranitidine
5. Antiarrhythmic drugs, e.g., flecainide
6. Antihypertensive medications, e.g., enalapril
7. Antidepressants, e.g., tricyclic antidepressants
8. Anticonvulsants, e.g., gabapentin, carbamazepine, and primidone

Central Disorders Causing Dizziness

1. Brainstem stroke or TIA
2. Parkinsonism
3. CNS tumors
4. CNS infections

5. Head trauma including postconcussion syndrome
6. Vertebrobasilar migraine
7. Multiple sclerosis

Peripheral Disorders Causing Dizziness

1. *Aural Causes*

   (a) BPPV
   (b) Ménière's disease
   (c) Vestibular neuronitis/viral labyrinthitis
   (d) Otitis and inner ear infections
   (e) Superior semicircular canal dehiscence syndrome
   (f) Otosclerosis

2. *Non-aural/Systemic Causes*

   (a) Orthostatic hypotension, cardiac arrhythmias, aortic stenosis, cardiomyopathy, anemia, dehydration, and hypoglycemia

References

1. Baloh RW, Kerber KA. Clinical neurophysiology of the vestibular system. In: Contemporary neurology series. 4th ed. New York: Oxford University Press; 2011.
2. Kutz Jr JW. The dizzy patient. Med Clin North Am. 2010;94(5):989–1002.
3. Bradley JG, Davis KA. Orthostatic hypotension. Am Fam Physician. 2003;68(12):2393–8.
4. Fife TD. Positional dizziness. Continuum (Minneap Minn). 2012;18(5 Neuro-otology):1060–85.

Chapter 4
Facial Weakness (Bell's Palsy)

Bell's palsy is an idiopathic facial paralysis that results from acquired cranial nerve VII (facial nerve) dysfunction. It usually presents with a sudden onset unilateral inability to move facial muscles on the affected side, although it is mostly self-limiting.

Peripheral facial nerve dysfunction presents as facial muscle paralysis, with or without loss of taste sensation on the anterior two-thirds of the tongue. It may be progressive, reaching its most debilitating state within 3 weeks from the onset. The diagnosis of Bell's palsy becomes unlikely if even minute levels of facial function do not return in 3 to 4 months. About 80–85 % of patients have spontaneous and complete recovery within 3 months, with a variable degree of residual deficits in the rest [1].

Stabilize the Patient

ABCs

1. Assess the airway and breathing rate, and look for signs of respiratory distress. Most patients will be stable.
2. Check the vital signs and assess if the patient is hemodynamically stable. Place the patient on a cardiac monitor and pulse oximeter. Most patients will be stable.

A.Q. Rana, J.A. Morren, *Neurological Emergencies in Clinical Practice,* DOI 10.1007/978-1-4471-5191-3_4, © Springer-Verlag London 2013

Focused History

1. Ask about the presenting symptoms, time of onset, and if progressive or not. There may be no antecedent symptoms of a viral syndrome like an upper respiratory tract infection.
2. Ask questions to rule out any other causes of the presenting symptoms especially other deficits suggestive of stroke.

Focused Exam

1. Assess language function. Check for naming, repetition, fluency, and comprehension.
2. Evaluate cranial nerve function including visual fields, lifting eyebrows and frowning, and nasolabial fold symmetry. Assess ability to blow cheeks out, seal lips, and whistle. Check strength of eyelid closure and assess hearing. Patients have ipsilateral eyebrow sagging or inability to generate wrinkles, inability to close eyes completely, and loss of nasolabial fold with drooping (and/or drooling) at corner of the mouth. Depending on the severity and extent of the lesion, patients may have hyperacusis ipsilaterally. A key finding is weakness affecting the upper face (including forehead) which is usually spared in an upper motor neuron-type facial palsy.

Identify the Underlying Cause

Take Further History

Ask about any additional symptoms, such as reduction in lacrimation, hyperacusis, and loss of taste sensation or recent history of head trauma (a rare cause). Decreased lacrimation, hyperacusis, and loss of taste on anterior two-thirds of tongue may be associated symptoms which provide information on the severity of the illness including the degree of proximal extension of the facial nerve lesion.

Do Further Examination

A complete neurological examination should be done. This includes testing mental status, other cranial nerves, muscle tone and power, muscle bulk and adventitious movements, deep tendon reflexes, plantar responses, coordination with station and gait assessment, as well as sensory examination of all modalities. Other non-cranial nerve deficits may indicate a central etiology like stroke.

Do Investigations

1. Usually no investigations are necessary if the clinical picture is consistent with diagnosis of Bell's palsy.
2. Electrodiagnostic tests such as NCS/EMG including blink reflex testing can help to confirm the diagnosis and indicate severity but are usually not required. Imaging studies are not required either. They can sometimes help to rule out other causes such as stroke, acoustic neuromas, or other focal mass lesions if the diagnosis is questionable. As most cases are self-limiting, further advanced diagnostic tests are usually unnecessary.

Treat the Underlying Cause

Treatment varies, depending on the individual and the severity of the illness. Mild cases may not require treatment as they subside generally within 2 weeks. In other cases, treatment include:

1. Prednisone (60 mg daily for 5 days, then decreased by 10 mg daily for a total of 10 days of treatment) can help to reduce inflammation. In diabetics, prednisone may be dosed at 30 mg/day for 2–3 days. Steroid usage is now a level A recommendation [2].
2. Acyclovir (400 mg three times daily for 5 days) can be prescribed for possible viral causes, but its added benefit is uncertain [2, 3].

3. Artificial eye drops (Lacri-lube®) can used to maintain lubrication during the day, and an eye patch can be applied at night time to avoid corneal ulceration, a dreaded complication.

Discussion

A serious complication to be wary of is corneal damage because of excessive dryness resulting in corneal ulceration due to inability to completely close the eye on the affected side. As such, proper eye care is an important part of treatment.

References

1. Finsterer J. Management of peripheral facial nerve palsy. Eur Arch Otorhinolaryngol. 2008;265(7):743–52.
2. Gronseth GS, Paduga R, American Academy of Neurology. Evidence-based guideline update: steroids and antivirals for Bell palsy: report of the Guideline Development Subcommittee of the American Academy of Neurology. Neurology. 2012; 79(22):2209–13.
3. Lampert L, Wong YJ. Combined antiviral-corticosteroid therapy for Bell palsy yields inconclusive benefit. J Am Dent Assoc. 2012; 143(1):57–8.

Chapter 5
Giant Cell Arteritis/Temporal Arteritis

Patients with giant cell arteritis are usually above the age of 50 and present with new onset headache which is due to an idiopathic inflammatory process involving the cranial arteries.

To better differentiate GCA from another form of vasculitis, at least three of the following five criteria must be present:

1. Age at disease onset of 50 years or older: development of symptoms or findings beginning at 50 years or older
2. New headache: new onset of, or new type of, localized pain in the head
3. Temporal artery abnormality: temporal artery tenderness to palpation or decreased pulsation, unrelated to arteriosclerosis of cervical arteries
4. Elevated ESR: an ESR of 50 mm/h or more by the Westergren method
5. Abnormal artery biopsy: biopsy specimen with artery showing vasculitis characterized by a predominance of mononuclear cell infiltration or granulomatous inflammation, usually with multinucleated giant cells [1]

Symptoms and signs:

1. Constitutional symptoms.
2. Headache: intense and mostly unilateral over one temple but can be bilateral, throbbing, boring, or burning, with an occasional stabbing sensation across the temporal area.

A.Q. Rana, J.A. Morren, *Neurological Emergencies in Clinical Practice*, DOI 10.1007/978-1-4471-5191-3_5, © Springer-Verlag London 2013

Aggravating factors: contact while combing hair or resting head on a pillow, opening the mouth, lying flat, and stooping

Alleviating factors: moving to an upright position and applying pressure over the common carotid artery

3. Facial swelling and red nodules over the temporal area can occur.

4. Visual symptoms: transient blurring of vision, diplopia, ophthalmoplegia, and even ptosis may develop 4–6 months after the onset of headaches. *There is a potential risk of loss of vision due to anterior ischemic optic neuropathy (AION)*, which occurs in 10–15 % of untreated or undertreated patients due to involvement of the ophthalmic artery [2].

5. Before major symptoms appear, pain may present in the teeth, zygoma, jaw, tongue, ear, nuchal, or occipital area due to involvement of other arteries such as external carotid artery and internal or external maxillary arteries. Other major vessels such as coronary arteries and branches of aorta may be involved as well.

Stabilize the Patient

ABCs

1. Assess the airway and breathing rate, and look for signs of respiratory distress.

2. Check the vital signs and assess if the patient is hemodynamically stable. Place the patient on a cardiac monitor and pulse oximeter. Most patients will be stable.

Focused History

1. Take a focused history of the presenting symptom and onset.

2. Ask questions to rule out other potentially serious causes of headaches such as acute onset of extremely severe headache, change in mental status, and focal motor or sensory symptoms.

Identify the Underlying Cause

Take Further History

1. Ask about the location and severity of headaches. Headaches from giant cell arteritis are usually of recent onset, start gradually, and become continuous daily precipitant headaches. Throbbing, sharp, stabbing exacerbations, and scalp tenderness may be present. Patients may also complain of being unable to comb hair due to exquisite scalp tenderness.
2. Ask about systemic symptoms such as myalgias, difficulty going up the stairs due to pain, malaise, low-grade fever, night sweats, jaw claudication, weight loss, and anorexia. Jaw claudication is a very useful diagnostic clue. About 50 % of patients with giant cell arteritis have polymyalgia rheumatica and complain about shoulder and hip girdle stiffness and pain.

Do Further Examination

1. A complete neurological examination should be done. This includes testing mental status, cranial nerves, muscle bulk, tone, power, adventitious movements, deep tendon reflexes, plantar responses, coordination with station and gait assessment, as well as sensory examination of all modalities.
2. Check visual acuity, visual fields, fundi, and palpate temporal arteries as they may be enlarged, hardened/cord-like, tender, or pulseless.

Do Investigations

1. ESR
   ESR by Westergren's method is above 50 in about 80 % of patients and above 100 in about 40 % of the patients. A normal ESR does not rule out temporal arteritis.
2. Check hemoglobin and hematocrit. Anemia is common.

3. CRP and Fibrinogen
   CRP and fibrinogen are markers of inflammation and may be elevated.
4. Temporal Artery Biopsy
   The patient should be scheduled for a temporal artery biopsy on an urgent basis. Because involvement of the temporal artery may be patchy, biopsy results may be falsely negative. If the suspicion is high, and the initial biopsy is negative, a biopsy of the contralateral side should be done.

Treat the Underlying Cause

Because of the risk of vision loss in untreated patients, giant cell arteritis is an emergency. If the diagnosis is strongly suspected, do the following:

1. Immediately start 60 mg of prednisone with a slow tapering schedule. Rapid improvement should occur and the ESR should return to normal. *Steroid treatment should not be delayed while waiting for temporal artery biopsy* [3].
2. Use a long-term maintenance dose of 10–20 mg of prednisone for 6 months to a year. Cyclophosphamide may be used for steroid sparing.
3. GI prophylaxis, blood glucose monitoring (especially in diabetics) should be started and the risk of side-effects including avascular necrosis of bones should be discussed with the patient.
4. Give calcium and vitamin D +/– a bisphosphonate like alendronate sodium.

Discussion

Anterior Ischemic Optic Neuropathy (AION)

The main complication in untreated patients is permanent loss of vision. Granulomatous inflammation can affect the temporal, ophthalmic and short posterior ciliary arteries and can result in anterior ischemic optic neuropathy. On biopsy, inflammatory infiltrates of lymphocytes and giant cells are seen involving the internal elastic lamina, although there may be patchy involvement with skip lesions.

References

1. Hunder GG, Bloch DA, Michel BA, Stevens MB, Arend WP, Calabrese LH, et al. The American College of Rheumatology 1990 criteria for the classification of giant cell arteritis. Arthritis Rheum. 1990;33:1122–8.
2. Gonzalez-Gay MA, Blanco R, Rodriquez-Valverde V, Martinez-Taboada VM, Delgado-Rodriguez M, Figueroa M, et al. Permanent visual loss and cerebrovascular accidents in giant cell arteritis: predictors and response to treatment. Arthritis Rheum. 1998;41:1497–504.
3. Gonzalez-Gay MA, Martinez-Dubois C, Agudo M, Pompei O, Blanco R, Llorca J. Giant cell arteritis: epidemiology, diagnosis, and management. Curr Rheumatol Rep. 2010;12(6):436–42.

Chapter 6
Guillain-Barré Syndrome

Guillain-Barré syndrome (GBS) is an acute inflammatory demyelinating polyradiculoneuropathy due to immune-mediated attack against surface antigens in peripheral nerve myelin sheaths [1].

Patients usually present with a history of rapidly progressive symmetrical ascending weakness. This starts in lower extremities initially and then may progress to involve the trunk, upper extremities, respiratory muscles, and cranial muscles. Paresthesias and other sensory symptoms as well as back pain may occur early in many patients [2].

Stabilize the Patient

ABCs

1. Assess the airway and breathing rate, and look for signs of respiratory distress. *Arterial blood gases may be normal early in respiratory muscle weakness, but early intubation favors a better prognosis*, so the decision to intubate and ventilate should be made when any of the following occur:

   (a) Clinical signs of respiratory compromise (e.g., tachypnea, use of accessory muscles)
   (b) Significant bulbar weakness
   (c) Vital capacity less than 20 ml/kg, maximum expiratory pressure less than 40 cmH$_2$O, and maximum inspiratory pressure weaker than −30 cmH$_2$O [3]

A.Q. Rana, J.A. Morren, *Neurological Emergencies in Clinical Practice*, DOI 10.1007/978-1-4471-5191-3_6, © Springer-Verlag London 2013

2. Check vital signs and assess if the patient is hemodynami-cally stable. Place the patient on a cardiac monitor and pulse oximeter. Provide I.V. fluids and pressors if required, as autonomic instability and cardiac arrhythmias are not uncommon.

Focused History

Enquire about presenting symptoms and onset. Patients usually have a history of rapidly progressive symmetrical ascending weakness.

Identify the Underlying Cause

Take Further History

1. Ask about the onset and progression of weakness. The first symptoms can be tingling or paresthesias in the lower extremities. Weakness affects the lower extremities ini-tially; sometimes proximal muscles are affected first. The maximum deficit occurs within 4 weeks and then plateaus. Lower back pain from radicular inflammation is common.
2. Ask about antecedent infections within the last 4–6 weeks. Approximately 2/3 of patients have a history of recent upper respiratory tract infection, gastroenteritis, immunization, or surgery. Infections preceding GBS include *Campylobacter jejuni* gastroenteritis (which is associated with a poor out-come), mycoplasma pneumonia, influenza, CMV and EBV.
3. Ask details about back pain and bowel and bladder symp-toms, to rule out any spinal cord or cauda equina pathologies.

Do Further Examination

1. A complete neurological examination should be done. This includes testing mental status, cranial nerves, muscle bulk, tone, power, adventitious movements, deep tendon

reflexes, plantar responses, coordination with station and gait assessment, as well as sensory examination of all modalities.

2. Cranial Nerve Assessment

   (a) 50 % develop bilateral facial weakness.
   (b) Ophthalmoplegia can occur.

3. Motor and Sensory Assessment

   (a) Lower extremity hypotonia and weakness
   (b) Mild sensory abnormalities: decreased vibration and position sense.

   NO sensory level, but may have low back pain

   (c) Lower extremity hypo- or areflexia
   (d) Flexor plantar responses

   - Contrast this with spinal cord compression where patients usually have spasticity, hyperreflexia, extensor plantar responses, more pronounced sensory abnormalities with a sensory level and back pain

Neck flexor and infraspinatus weakness most strongly correlates with diaphragmatic weakness from phrenic nerve involvement. Generally, patients who are unable to count to 20 in a single exhaled of breath are likely having significant respiratory compromise.

Do Further Investigations

1. Routine Labs
   CBC, electrolytes, calcium, AST, ALT, INR, flu testing, serology for *Campylobacter jejuni* ± specific virology as indicated.
2. MRI of the Spine
   Required to *rule out spinal cord pathology* if patients have spasticity, extensor plantar responses, or a sensory level. MRI may also rule out cauda equina pathology in a patient with lower extremity hypotonia, areflexia, and flexor

plantar responses (also typical for GBS). In GBS, lumbar nerve roots may enhance in a contrasted study.

3. Lumbar Puncture

   If there is no suspicion of cord compression, CSF analysis is required. Typically CSF has increased protein and a normal cell count (albumino-cytological dissociation), although some patients may have 10–50 cells/mm^3 with a lymphocytic predominance.

4. Nerve Conduction Studies

   Typically nerve conduction studies show prolonged F waves, absent H-reflexes, focal or segmental slowing, conduction block, reduced conduction velocities, prolonged distal latencies, and temporal dispersion of motor responses. Reduced compound motor action potential (CMAP) amplitude and denervation changes on needle electrode examination indicate axonal damage which predicts a poorer prognosis.

Treat the Underlying Cause

1. Respiratory Muscle Weakness

   Early intubation is very important and leads to earlier extubation and a better prognosis. Intubation should not be guided by pulse oximetry or arterial blood gases, which are often normal until severe respiratory distress occurs. Nonetheless, intubation should be performed if: $pO_2 < 70$, $pCO_2 > 50$, and $pH < 7.35$. Vital capacity (VC) should be measured at least every 4–6 h if the patient is not intubated and every 12 h if intubated.

   Guidelines for ventilation are:

   (a) Avoid succinylcholine – this agent can precipitate lethal hyperkalemia particularly in the context of severe disease with denervation.

   (b) Synchronized intermittent mandatory ventilation (SIMV) mode at 8–10 breaths per minute. If there is severe respiratory muscle weakness, use the assist control (AC) mode to provide complete ventilatory support until some recovery occurs.

(c) Tidal volume of 10–15 ml/kg ideal body weight.

(d) Positive end expiratory pressure (PEEP) of 5–10 cmH_2O to prevent atelectasis. Excess PEEP should be avoided to allow venous return and minimize risk of autonomic decompensation.

To reduce aspiration and pneumonia risk, the head of the bed should be elevated, chest physiotherapy should be done regularly, and appropriate nutritional support should be given.

2. Continuous Cardiac Monitoring
   GBS patients are at risk of autonomic instability and cardiac arrhythmia.

3. Immune-Modulating Therapy.
   Intravenous immunoglobulin and plasma exchange/plasmapheresis have been shown to have similar efficacy in the management of GBS [4, 5].

   Intravenous immunoglobulin (IVIG): The dose is 0.4 g/kg/day for 5 days. IVIG reduces the time to recovery and decreases the need for mechanical ventilation. *IgA levels should be checked in all patients before starting IVIG* because of the increased risk of anaphylaxis in patients with IgA deficiency. Side effects of IVIG include headache, renal failure, allergic reactions, aseptic meningitis, hemolytic anemia, and hypercoagulability-related complications like DVT and stroke.

   Plasma exchange: This is performed on alternate days for a total of five treatments and is more effective when given early. Plasma exchange decreases mechanical ventilation time, hospital stay, and time to walking again and leads to better muscle strength recovery. Side effects include infections, arrhythmias, hypotension, bleeding, and hypocalcaemia.

4. Tracheostomy
   If patients are intubated for 2+ weeks, tracheostomy should be considered.

5. Pain control, DVT and GI Prophylaxis

Discussion

Clinical Variants of GBS

1. Miller Fisher Syndrome
   This is characterized by ophthalmoparesis, ataxia, and areflexia. It is often associated with IgG antibody to ganglioside GQ1b and prior *Campylobacter jejuni* infection.
2. Acute Axonal Variant
   This variant has a poor prognosis and manifests as early respiratory muscle involvement, quadriplegia, and other bulbar dysfunction. It may also be associated with *Campylobacter jejuni* infection. Patients may have an increased titer of anti-GM1 antibodies.

Differential Diagnosis of GBS

1. Spinal Cord Lesion
   Patients usually have prominent sensory abnormalities, a sensory level, spasticity, hyperreflexia, clonus, and extensor plantar response and may have bowel and bladder dysfunction.
2. Cauda Equina Lesion
   Sensory abnormalities consistent with "saddle anesthesia," urinary dysfunction, hypotonia and hyporeflexia in lower extremities, and flexor plantar responses.
3. Botulism
   Botulism causes a descending paralysis, in contrast to the ascending paralysis of GBS.
4. Tick Paralysis
   CSF protein is usually normal, in contrast to the elevated levels in GBS.
5. Other Conditions
   Lyme disease, saxitoxin, tetrodotoxin, and ciguatera poisoning from shellfish, hypokalemia, hypophosphatemia, porphyria, hexane, arsenic, lead, and thallium poisoning.

References

1. Yuki N. Guillain-Barré syndrome and anti-ganglioside antibodies: a clinician-scientist's journey. Proc Jpn Acad Ser B Phys Biol Sci. 2012;88(7):299–326.
2. Yuki N, Hartung HP. Guillain-Barré syndrome. N Engl J Med. 2012;366(24):2294–304.
3. Rabinstein AA, Wijdicks EF. Warning signs of imminent respiratory failure in neurological patients. Semin Neurol. 2003;23(1): 97–104.
4. Van Der Meche FG, Schmitz PI. A randomized trial comparing intravenous immune globulin and plasma exchange in Guillain-Barré syndrome. Dutch Guillain-Barré Study Group. N Engl J Med. 1992;326:1123–9.
5. Hughes RA, Wijdicks EF, Barohn R, Benson E, Cornblath DR, Hahn AF, et al. Practice parameter: immunotherapy for Guillain-Barré syndrome: report of the Quality Standards Subcommittee of the American Academy of Neurology. Neurology. 2003;61: 736–40.

References

Chapter 7
Headache

The most important step in the evaluation of headaches is to rule out underlying potentially serious secondary causes such as subarachnoid hemorrhage, meningitis, epidural or subdural hematoma, cerebral venous sinus thrombosis, pseudotumor cerebri, giant cell arteritis, and intracranial mass lesion.

History and physical examination provide very important clues to the diagnosis of these conditions. Once the above-mentioned secondary causes of headaches are ruled out, the primary headaches are classified mainly into migraine, tension-type headaches, and trigeminal autonomic cephalgias (which include cluster headaches and paroxysmal hemicrania, among others) and can be managed in the outpatient clinic once the patient is stable.

Stabilize the Patient

ABCs

1. Assess the airway and breathing rate, and look for signs of respiratory distress. Most patients presenting primarily with headaches are stable. If there is a decreased level of consciousness (especially if GCS is less than or equal to eight), the patient may need to be intubated first.
2. Check the vital signs and assess if the patient is hemodynamically stable. Provide fluids if needed. Place the patient

A.Q. Rana, J.A. Morren, *Neurological Emergencies in Clinical Practice,* DOI 10.1007/978-1-4471-5191-3_7, © Springer-Verlag London 2013

in a quiet and dimly lit room if possible and on a cardiac monitor and pulse oximeter.

Focused History

1. Ask about presenting symptoms and onset.
2. Ask if there is any history of head injury, the nature and extent of the head injury, and whether there was any decline in the level of consciousness.
3. Ask if the patient is a known headache sufferer or if the onset of headaches is new.
4. If the patient has a history of frequent headaches, ask if this headache is similar to previous ones, more intense, or entirely different than previous headaches. *A sudden onset of extremely severe headache is suggestive of subarachnoid hemorrhage.* These patients may not have any previous history of headaches.
5. Ask if there is any history of fever in last 24 h. Determine if there is any change in mental status. *Headache with fever and change in mental status is suggestive of meningitis; lumbar puncture is required.*

Focused Examination

1. Note any evidence of trauma or infection in sinuses, nose, throat, neck, and ear canals.
2. Check for papilledema, subhyaloid hemorrhages (which are boat-shaped hemorrhages seen in the retina in cases of subarachnoid hemorrhage), and pupil response. Horner's syndrome may be seen with cluster headache. *A unilateral dilated fixed pupil with a decreased level of consciousness may be sign of herniation* such as can be seen in epidural and subdural hematoma, stroke with cerebral edema, and focal mass lesions. *This is a neurological emergency.*
3. Look for lateralizing signs on motor testing and extensor plantar responses.

4. Assess neck stiffness and look for meningeal signs. Meningeal signs have low sensitivity and specificity. Neck stiffness with extension and flexion but normal rotation is a more reliable sign of meningitis. Also, meningismus is not specific to infection, but can be seen in subarachnoid hemorrhage.

   Brudzinski's sign is present if passive flexion of the patient's neck by the examiner results in flexion of the lower extremities.

   Kernig's sign is present if, with hip and knee in flexion, passive extension of the knee is restricted by hamstring spasm and/or pain.

Initial Investigations

1. CT Scan of the Head
   This is required if any lateralizing signs are present or if subarachnoid hemorrhage is suspected.
2. Lumbar Puncture
   This is required if meningitis or subarachnoid hemorrhage is suspected and the CT scan is normal. *Only perform a lumbar puncture if the CT scan is negative for any space-occupying lesions.*

Identify the Underlying Cause

Take Further History

1. Ask what the patient was doing at the time of headache onset and whether any neck pain accompanied headache.
2. Ask about any alteration in level of consciousness. Intracranial bleeding can be associated with transient loss of consciousness.
3. Ask about other symptoms of increased intracranial pressure such as nausea or vomiting especially with lying. Determine if the patient has visual symptoms, speech alteration, weakness, or numbness.

4. Headache upon awakening is suggestive of increased intracranial pressure as can be seen with a space-occupying lesion.
5. Ask about recent ear, nose, throat, and sinus infections that might have developed into an abscess or increased the risk for cerebral venous sinus thrombosis.
6. In elderly patients, consider giant cell arteritis which is associated with scalp tenderness and jaw and tongue claudication and with systemic symptoms such as fever, chills, rashes, night sweats, weight loss, and myalgias with hip and shoulder girdle stiffness. (Please see Chap. 5.)
7. Pseudotumor cerebri or benign intracranial hypertension is associated with weight gain and transient visual obscurations. Permanent vision loss can occur if not treated. (Please see Chap. 15.)
8. Ask about the nature and severity of headaches and whether they are unilateral, generalized, switching sides, or positional.
9. Ask about features suggestive of migraine. These include sensitivity to light, noise, or smells; the presence of an aura; nausea or vomiting; and scalp hypersensitivity or allodynia. There may be aggravating factors such as sleep deprivation, hunger, physical exertion, menstrual periods, stress, chocolate, caffeine, and (possibly) foods rich in tyramine such as cheese and red wine. There is often a family history of migraine.
10. Cluster headaches are periorbital/temporal pain associated with a sense of restlessness associated with ipsilateral conjunctival injection, lacrimation, or rhinorrhea. They tend to recur at the same time of night (alarm clock headaches), lasting 15–180 min with recurrence from every other day to as frequent as eight times per day. Other trigeminal autonomic cephalgias have similar autonomic symptoms but distinctive durations and frequencies.
11. Trigeminal neuralgia presents as a sharp jabbing electric shock-like pain and is often exacerbated with laughing, talking, chewing, or brushing teeth. There may be associated tender points on the face or head and neck area.
12. Temporomandibular joint problems may cause headaches and may be associated with teeth grinding (bruxism).

13. Snoring with an unrefreshed feeling in the mornings and daytime sleepiness may indicate obstructive sleep apnea.
14. The excessive use of analgesics can cause analgesic rebound headaches/medication overuse headache.
15. Ask about relieving factors, medications used for break-through headaches, and if any prophylaxis has been tried so far.

Do Further Examination

1. A complete neurological examination should be done. This includes testing mental status, cranial nerves, muscle bulk, tone, power, adventitious movements, deep tendon reflexes, plantar responses, coordination with station and gait assessment, as well as sensory examination of all modalities.
2. Palpate for temporal artery tenderness/hardening.

Further Investigations

1. A CT scan of the head is indicated in the following scenarios:

   (a) History of acute onset of extremely severe headache
   (b) Headache different than previous headaches
   (c) Change in mental status, papilledema, and focal motor and/or sensory signs
   (d) Suspected meningitis
   (e) Suspicion of intracerebral or cerebellar hemorrhage, infarct, mass, or history of anticoagulant use
   (f) Other signs of increased intracranial pressure
   (g) Patients requiring lumbar puncture
   (h) Significant head trauma, skull fracture, penetrating head injury, or Glasgow Coma Scale of less than 9 (see Chap. 1)

2. Other investigations depend on the suspected underlying cause of headache:

   (a) *Infection*: A CBC is indicated with ESR, CRP, lumbar puncture for CSF analysis – including cell count, protein, glucose, Gram stain, fungal stains, culture and sensitivities, and +/− virology.

(b) *Focal mass lesions (brain tumor or abscess)*: A brain MRI with and without contrast is required.

(c) *Giant cell arteritis*: Check ESR, CRP, and fibrinogen. Also check PT, INR, and serum chemistry in case the patient needs surgical intervention.

(d) *Subarachnoid hemorrhage*: A CT scan is required. If the CT scan is normal, a lumbar puncture is mandatory. *If indicative, a cerebral angiogram with neurosurgical and radiology consultation is required.*

(e) *Pseudotumor cerebri*: A lumbar puncture for opening pressure is required (see Chap. 15). *A CT scan must be done before lumbar puncture to rule out focal mass lesions.*

Differential Diagnosis

Consider headaches in terms of primary and secondary causes. The secondary causes often require more urgent treatment or intervention and so are discussed first.

1. Secondary Causes of Headache

(a) *Subarachnoid Hemorrhage (SAH)*
Immediate diagnosis and treatment is necessary because about 20 % rebleed within 2 weeks and 35 % over the first 4 weeks if the aneurysm is untreated. Up to 65 % of patients who rebleed will die [1].

Suggestive symptoms and signs:

1. Acute onset of extremely severe headache
2. Change in mental status
3. Subhyaloid hemorrhages (which are boat-shaped hemorrhages seen in the retina)
4. Meningeal signs
5. Photophobia

Causes:

1. Trauma
2. Aneurysm

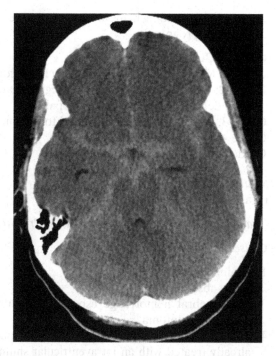

FIGURE. 7.1 Non-contrasted head CT scan with subarachnoid hemorrhage. Hyperdense blood mostly in the suprasellar cistern, prepontine cistern, and Sylvian fissures (Courtesy of Dr. I. Haq)

3. Arteriovenous malformations
4. Other vascular pathologies

CT scan findings (Fig. 7.1):

1. Hyperdensity in the major fissures, sulci, or around the brainstem.
2. In 5–10 % of patients, the CT scan is normal; in these cases, lumbar puncture is required.

CSF findings:

1. Xanthochromia
2. Increased red blood cells, usually in the thousands, without any decline from tube 1 to tube 4 (in contrast to a traumatic lumbar puncture where there are more red cells in the earlier tubes)

Hunt and Hess grading helps in management decisions and predicts prognosis:

Grade 0: Unruptured aneurysm
Grade 1: Minor headache and mild nuchal rigidity
Grade 2: Severe headache, nuchal rigidity, and no focal deficits except cranial nerve palsies
Grade 3: Lethargy, confusion, or mild focal deficit
Grade 4: Stupor and hemiparesis
Grade 5: Coma or decerebrate rigidity

(b) *Meningitis or Encephalitis*
Please see Chap. 9 for details.

(c) *Headaches Due to Increased Intracranial Pressure*

Causes:

1. Brain tumor
2. Brain abscess
3. Intracerebral hemorrhage especially subdural or epidural hematoma
4. *Acute hydrocephalus*: usually occurs in patients already treated with an intraventricular shunt who develop obstruction or malfunction of the shunt. *Emergency ventricular drainage is required.*

Symptoms and signs:

1. Drowsiness, slow thinking, and confusion
2. Focal motor and/or sensory signs
3. Papilledema
4. Nausea and vomiting
5. Seizures
6. History of aural and sinus infections, leukocytosis, and fever

(d) *Headaches Due to Intracranial Hypertension*
The main condition to consider is:
Benign intracranial hypertension (pseudotumor cerebri) (see Chap. 15)

(e) *Giant Cell Arteritis*
Please see Chap. 5.

(f) *Arteriovenous Malformation*
These vary in size and are present at birth but may be asymptomatic until adolescence or later. They may cause headaches, intracerebral hemorrhages, seizures, or progressive neurological deficits.

(g) *Neuralgias*
Causes of facial pain and headaches include:

1. *Trigeminal neuralgia*: characterized by unilateral, brief, episodic, recurrent, electric shock-like lancinating pain in the distribution of the trigeminal nerve, usually the maxillary (V2) and mandibular (V3) branches. Pain may radiate to the ophthalmic (V1) branch late in the disease. This rarely begins before age 50 unless the patient has multiple sclerosis. The pain is exacerbated by touching trigger points or by laughing, talking, chewing, eating, or brushing teeth. Patients may develop an avoidance of these activities, which is a diagnostic clue. *An MRI is indicated to rule out brainstem lesions or pontine demyelination in young patients.*

2. *Glossopharyngeal neuralgia*: similar to trigeminal neuralgia except the pain is localized to the pharynx and tonsils and is triggered by yawning, swallowing, and eating.

3. *Occipital neuralgia*: causes pain in the upper neck and occipital area.

(h) *Headaches Due to Spontaneous Intracranial Hypotension or Posttrauma/Intervention*
These headaches are caused by leakage of CSF through a defect in the arachnoid +/− dura mater.

Causes:

1. Lumbar puncture (the most common)
2. Primary intracranial hypotension/occult spinal dural leak

3. CSF rhinorrhea or otorrhea
4. Malfunctioning ventricular shunt

Symptoms and signs:

1. Begins within hours to days after lumbar puncture and may last several weeks.
2. Dull, deep aching, or throbbing; bifrontal or suboccipital.
3. May be associated with neck stiffness.
4. The headache begins as soon as the patient assumes an upright position and improves with return to the supine position.
5. Shaking the head or coughing may exacerbate the headache.

MRI findings:
Pachymeningeal/meningeal enhancement

(i) *Hypertensive Encephalopathy*
Hypertension usually does not cause headaches unless the blood pressure is very high (see below).

Symptoms and signs:

1. Systolic pressure >220 mmHg and diastolic pressure >120 mmHg
2. Occipital or frontal headache and throbbing
3. Nausea and vomiting
4. Focal neurological signs
5. May have papilledema, decreased level of consciousness, and cardiovascular changes

2. Primary Causes of Headaches
If none of the secondary causes are suspected, and the patient is a known headache sufferer, then the headache may be due to primary causes including migraine, tension-type headaches, cluster headaches, or other trigeminal autonomic cephalgias as well as other miscellaneous causes [2]:

(a) *Migraine with or Without Aura*

Symptoms and signs:

1. Usually throbbing in nature.
2. Unilateral or switching sides.
3. History of photophobia, sonophobia, or sensitivity to smells.
4. Nausea and vomiting.
5. May have triggers such as exertion, fatigue, menstrual periods, and (possibly) foods rich in tyramine such as cheese and red wine.
6. May or may not have visual aura or paresthesias/skin sensory auras.
7. Females are affected more than males.

(b) *Tension-Type Headaches*
These are the most prevalent type of headaches presenting in the emergency room.

Symptoms and signs:

1. Usually described as a tightening, aching, or band-like sensation
2. Often generalized predominantly involving occipital or frontal area
3. Usually starting late in the morning and worsening in the afternoon
4. May have episodic on top of chronic tension-type headaches

(c) *Cluster Headaches and Other trigeminal Autonomic Cephalgia*

Symptoms and signs:

1. May be periorbital with ipsilateral lacrimation or nasal congestion/rhinorrhea with episodes lasting 15–180 min.
2. Often occur at the same time every day (alarm clock headaches) or after the patient goes to sleep.

3. May have ipsilateral Horner's syndrome and conjunctival flushing/injection.
4. Usually occur daily from 3 weeks to 3 months and
   then go into remission.
5. May be exacerbated by alcohol intake, also associated with smoking
6. Males are affected more than females.

Other trigeminal autonomic cephalgia have similar
autonomic features but distinctive durations and
frequencies.

Treat the Underlying Cause

Treatment of headache depends on the underlying cause (see
above).
1. Subarachnoid Hemorrhage
   An angiogram and consultation by neurosurgery and inter-
   ventional radiology are required. Treatment options include
   aneurysm clipping or coiling. *Fluid management is crucial*
   for the prevention of vasospasm, which occurs primarily
   between day 4 and 14. "Triple H" therapy includes induced
   hypertension, hypervolemia, and hemodilution. Nimodipine
   is also indicated for vasospasm prophylaxis and treatment.
2. Meningitis or Encephalitis
   See Chap. 9.
3. Elevated Intracranial Pressure
   An MRI with gadolinium is obtained and neurosurgical
   consultation is indicated for mass lesions.
4. Giant Cell Arteritis
   See Chap. 5.
5. Neuralgia (Trigeminal, Glossopharyngeal, or Occipital)
   Medical treatments include:

   (a) Carbamazepine 100–200 mg TID (the most effective).
       Oxcarbazepine is an alternative.
   (b) Phenytoin and chlorphenesin in refractory patients.
   (c) Can also try baclofen, gabapentin, or amitriptyline [3].

Surgical procedures include:

(a) Glycerol injection
(b) Radiofrequency rhizotomy
(c) Microvascular decompression of the trigeminal root (for trigeminal neuralgia)
(d) Nerve blocks for occipital neuralgia

6. Intracranial Hypotension or Post-lumbar Puncture Headache
   These headaches are often resistant to all forms of treatments. Bed rest, adequate hydration, caffeine, analgesics, and autologous epidural blood patch are advised.

7. Hypertensive Encephalopathy
   After a CT of the head has ruled out bleeding, an internal medicine consultation is required for the management of hypertension. Abrupt drops in blood pressure should be avoided to prevent cerebral dysautoregulation.

8. Migraine
   Treatment involves avoidance of exacerbating factors/triggers and the initiation of abortive and/or preventive treatments.

   Abortive treatments: acetaminophen +/− caffeine, aspirin, ibuprofen, naproxen, triptans, ketorolac, and ergotamine. Headache severity guides medication choice:

   - *Mild to moderate headache*:
     Treatment may include one the following:
     Sumatriptan nasal spray 20 mg, one spray in one nostril at onset, may repeat within 2–24 h, maximum dose of two sprays per day OR
     Zolmitriptan nasal spray 5 mg, may repeat once in 2 h, maximum dose of 10 mg/day OR
     Sumatriptan 6 mg subcutaneous, may repeat after 1 h, maximum dose of 12 mg/day (increasing use may not increase efficacy)
   - *Severe headache*:
     Prochlorperazine 10 mg I.V. or metoclopramide 10 mg I.M./I.V.
     plus dihydroergotamine (DHE), 1 mg I.M. or I.V.

over 2 min; DHE can be repeated every 1–2 h up to a maximum dose of 3 mg/day and 6 mg/week.
Dexamethasone (Decadron®) 4–10 mg I.V.
Ketorolac 15–30 mg I.V.

Prophylactic treatments: beta blockers, tricyclic antidepressants, topiramate, valproic acid, calcium channel blockers, pizotifen, and botulinum toxin injection

9. Tension-type headache:
   NSAIDs and tricyclic antidepressants.
   Narcotic analgesics should be avoided in these patients.

10. Cluster headaches:

    7–15 L/min of oxygen for 20 min plus SC sumatriptan 6 mg, or NS sumatriptan 20 mg, or NS zolmitriptan 5 mg
    +/− transitional steroid plus DHE treatment (allow 24 hrs after last triptan dose)

Discussion

For primary causes of headache, once the patient is stable, a referral to a neurologist for outpatient management should be made.

References

1. Wu TC, Tsui YK, Chen TY, Lin CJ, Wu TC, Tzeng WS. Rebleeding of aneurismal subarachnoid hemorrhage in computed tomography angiography: risk factor, rebleeding pattern, and outcome analysis. J Comput Assist Tomogr. 2012;36(1):103–8.
2. Silberstein SD, Lipton RB, Dodick DW, editors. Wolff's headache and other head pain. 8th ed. New York: Oxford University Press; 2008.
3. Gronseth G, Cruccu G, Alksne J, Argoff C, Brainin M, Burchiel K, Nurmikko T, Zakrzewska JM. Practice parameter: the diagnostic evaluation and treatment of trigeminal neuralgia (an evidence-based review): report of the Quality Standards Subcommittee of the American Academy of Neurology and the European Federation of Neurological Societies. Neurology. 2008;71(15):1183–90.

Chapter 8
Head Injury

The neurology or neurosurgical service is usually called if head injury is assessed as moderate to severe in degree. The Glasgow Coma Scale is pivotal in this evaluation. Timely assessment of these patients is necessary since they may have life-threatening injuries and if intervention is delayed, damage may be irreversible or fatal.

Stabilize the Patient

ABCs

1. If a cervical spine injury is suspected, the neck should be immobilized with a rigid cervical collar. *The head should not be moved until radiographic assessment is done to exclude cervical spine instability.*
2. Assess the airway and breathing rate, and look for signs of respiratory distress. If there is respiratory distress or a decreased level of consciousness (especially if GCS is less than or equal to 8), intubation and ventilation are required. If there is a suspicion of cervical spine injury, the intubation should be done with in-line stabilization without extension of the neck or by surgical airway if necessary.

    For suspected herniation or a Glasgow Coma Score of 8 or less, take measures to reduce elevated intracranial pressure:

A.Q. Rana, J.A. Morren, *Neurological Emergencies in Clinical Practice*, DOI 10.1007/978-1-4471-5191-3_8, © Springer-Verlag London 2013

    (a) Intubate under rapid induction.

    (b) Hyperventilate in IMV mode, 16–20 cycles per minute and tidal volume 10–15 ml/kg.

    (c) Elevate head of bed to 30°.

    (d) Target $paCO_2$ to 28–32 mmHg. (Caution: Over-aggressive hyperventilation with severe hypocapnia may cause excessive vasoconstriction resulting in cerebral ischemia and should be avoided.)

If there is no suggestion of increased ICP, no hyperventilation is required:

    (a) Target $paCO_2$ to 40 mmHg

    (b) Target paO_2 to 90 mmHg

3. Check the vital signs and assess if the patient is hemodynamically stable. Place the patient on a cardiac monitor and pulse oximeter. Maintain the circulation and monitor the blood pressure, pulse, cardiac rate, and rhythm continuously, and treat unstable vital signs and cardiac arrhythmias. Try to maintain a mean arterial pressure around 100 mmHg.

Focused History

Enquire about the circumstances surrounding and the extent of the injury from the available resources, including family members and paramedics, and review the emergency medical services sheet. It is important to formulate the mechanism of trauma (e.g., to focus on sites liable to coup/contrecoup injury).

Focused Exam

1. Inspect the head for signs of trauma (see further details in section "Identify the Underlying Cause").
2. Do a focused neurological exam (see Glasgow Coma Scale, Chap. 1). Include mental status assessment, observation of breathing pattern, pupil size and response, any eye

deviation, lateralizing signs, deep tendon reflexes, and plantar responses. (See section "Identify the Underlying Cause" for more detailed examination).
3. Perform cardiac and pulmonary auscultation.

STAT Labs and Treatments

1. Request C-spine x-rays to rule out a fracture from C1 to C7.
2. Start an I.V. line of normal saline.
3. Send blood work: CBC, hematocrit, electrolytes, glucose, creatinine, PT, INR, toxicology screen, and serum alcohol level. Check arterial blood gases. Type blood and hold in case transfusion is required.
4. Do a STAT CT scan of the head if the patient has a decline in level of consciousness, a depressed or penetrating skull fracture, vomiting, seizure, memory loss, signs of marked external trauma, significant headache, or a Glasgow Coma Score of 8 or less.

Identify the Underlying Cause

Take Further History

1. Ask about drug and alcohol use.
2. Ask further details about the injury, events, and course of the patient's condition since the injury. A progressive decline in level of consciousness may indicate an expanding subdural or epidural hematoma.

Do Further Examination

A complete neurological examination should be done. This includes testing mental status, cranial nerves, muscle bulk, tone, power, adventitious movements, deep tendon reflexes, plantar responses, coordination with station and gait assessment, as well as sensory examination of all modalities.

1. Mental Status

   Determine if the patient is awake and oriented or confused, lethargic, stuporous, or comatose.

2. Observe and Palpate for Signs of Skull Fracture

   Battle's sign: ecchymosis over the mastoid process.
   Raccoon eyes: ecchymosis around the periorbital area.
   CSF discharge: seen in the ears (CSF otorrhea) or nose (CSF rhinorrhea). CSF can be differentiated from mucous by its high glucose content on a dip stick. CSF forms a halo around blood when dropped on a cloth sheet.

3. Cranial Nerve Examination

   Include examination of fundus (exclude retinal hemorrhage, detachment); response to visual threat stimuli; pupillary size, shape, regularity, and reaction to light; extraocular movements; oculocephalic reflex (see Chap. 1 for details); vestibuloocular reflex (see Chap. 1 for details); corneal reflexes; facial asymmetry by grimace in response to pain or nasal tickle; and gag reflex. In intubated patients, the gag can be checked by manipulating the endotracheal tube and the cough reflex can be checked with deep suctioning. *A unilateral large fixed pupil with or without "down and out" eye deviation is a sign of cranial nerve III compression from uncal herniation and represents a neurological emergency.* (See Fig. 1.1.)

4. Motor and Sensory Examination

   Assess power in cooperative patients. In noncooperative patients, watch for lateralized spontaneous movements. If spontaneous movements are absent, observe the response to sternal rub, painful compression of nail beds, or supraorbital ridge pressure. Check the tone in both upper and lower limbs.

5. Deep Tendon Reflexes and Plantar Responses

   Asymmetry may indicate a focal deficit. An extensor plantar response is indicative of an upper motor neuron lesion.

6. Posturing

Assess posturing if the level of consciousness is decreased. Use painful stimuli.

Flexor response or decorticate posturing: flexion and adduction of upper extremities and extension of the lower extremities resulting from damage to the corticospinal tract at or above the level of the upper midbrain.

Extensor response or decerebrate posturing: extension and internal rotation of the upper extremities and extension of the lower extremities resulting from damage at or below the caudal midbrain-rostral pons level [1].

Do Further Investigations

1. CT Scan of Head

CT scan of the head, with and without bone windows, is assessed for skull fracture, subdural or epidural hematoma, subarachnoid hemorrhage, intracerebral hemorrhage, cerebral edema, obliteration of basal cisterns, and mass effect, including midline shift. If the CT scan shows any of the above abnormalities, admission to the ICU and neurosurgical consultation are indicated.

2. Lumbar Puncture

If the CT scan of head is normal but there is suspicion of subarachnoid hemorrhage, lumbar puncture is indicated for CSF analysis which may reveal xanthochromia and increased red blood cell count.

Treat the Underlying Cause

The management of head injury patients depends largely on the underlying cause (see below), but general management includes the following:

(a) Neurosurgical consultation for possible intervention.
(b) Patients may need intracranial pressure (ICP) monitoring if expanding mass lesion, intraventricular hemorrhage or acute hydrocephalus is present.
(c) Elevated ICP is treated with 20 % mannitol 1 g/kg titrated to serum osmolality. (Note: Steroids usually do not have a role in treating head injury patients.)
(d) Mean blood pressure should be monitored very closely.
(e) Fever should be treated aggressively.
(f) Only isotonic I.V. fluids should be given because hypotonic fluids might worsen cerebral edema.
(g) Provide DVT prophylaxis.
(h) Give GI protection with ranitidine 50 mg I.V. every 8 h or use of a proton pump inhibitor.
(i) Repeat a CT scan of the head in 24 h (or earlier if acute deterioration occurs).
(j) Place a Foley catheter for all cases of decreased level of consciousness.
(k) If there is a CSF leak, the patient may require a lumbar drain; CSF otorrhea or rhinorrhea requires surgical repair.

Treatment according to underlying cause:

1. Epidural Hematoma

   Epidural hematomas are of arterial source in about 85 % of cases and may be associated with a skull fracture. The most common source of bleeding in middle cranial fossa epidural hematomas is the middle meningeal artery. *Herniation and death can occur rapidly, so an urgent surgical evacuation is needed.*

   Symptoms and signs:

   (a) Ten to 27 % of patients have immediate loss of consciousness followed by a lucid interval and then recurrence of loss of consciousness.
   (b) May develop contralateral hemiparesis. (Note: Some develop ipsilateral hemiparesis due to compression of opposite cerebral peduncle on tentorial notch (Kernohan's notch). This is a false localizing sign.)

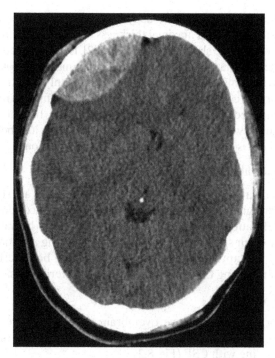

FIGURE 8.1 Non-contrasted head CT scan showing right frontal epidural hematoma (Courtesy of Dr. I. Haq)

    (c) Sixty percent have pupillary dilatation, which is ipsilateral 85 % of the time.

    (d) Headache, vomiting, seizures, and coma.

CT findings (Fig. 8.1):

    (a) Appear biconvex, have a uniform density, attenuation is high, and the edges are sharply defined.

    (b) They are contiguous with the inner table of skull.

    (c) Frequently accompanied by mass effect.

Treatment:

Any symptomatic epidural hematoma or acute epidural hematoma with an estimated volume more than 30 ml *should have urgent surgical evacuation*, regardless of GCS.

Such an indication is usually the case with epidural hematomas having a maximal thickness of 15 mm or more and/or a midline shift exceeding 5 mm [2]. Even small epidural hematomas with no herniation and minimal neurological symptoms may increase in size suddenly and require urgent craniotomy; therefore, surgical treatment is recommended. In the pediatric population, the threshold for surgery for epidural hematoma should be low because there is less room for the hematoma expansion.

2. Subdural Hematoma

The sources of bleeding in subdural hematomas are surface or bridging veins which are torn during an acceleration-deceleration movement of the head. Subdural hematomas may occur spontaneously in patients receiving anticoagulation therapy. Subdural hematomas may be interhemispheric, along the tentorium or in the posterior fossa.

CT findings:

(a) Appear concave over brain surface and are more diffuse, less uniform, and less dense because of mixing with CSF (Fig. 8.2)
(b) Density varies with age of hematoma:

Acute (1–3 days): hyperdense
Subacute (4 days to 3 weeks): isodense
Chronic (greater than 3 weeks): hypodense

Treatment:

Urgent neurosurgical intervention is needed for symptomatic subdural hematoma or any subdural hematoma with a midline shift more than or equal to 5 mm. It is also indicated for acute subdural hematomas exceeding 1 cm in maximal thickness regardless of GCS [3].
All acute subdural hematoma patients in coma (GCS score less than 9) should have intracranial pressure monitoring [4].
Small subdural hematomas need close observation.

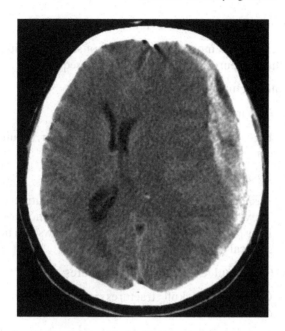

FIGURE 8.2 Non-contrasted head CT scan showing a left frontoparietal subdural hematoma with mass effect including midline shift (Courtesy of Dr. I. Haq)

3. Traumatic Intracerebral Hemorrhage

Traumatic intracerebral hemorrhage can occur following coup-contrecoup effects on the head.

CT findings:

(a) High density, usually in inferior frontal and temporal poles
(b) Less mass effect
(c) May evolve, enlarge, or coalesce with time

Treatment:

Close observation for at least 24 h is required. Repeat a CT scan and employ surgical decompression if there is a substantial chance of herniation.

4. Traumatic Subarachnoid Hemorrhage

Trauma is the most common cause of subarachnoid hemorrhage. Neurosurgical consultation is required.

5. Skull Fracture

(a) Linear skull fractures:

Eighty percent of skull fractures are linear, requiring a conservative approach.

(b) Basal skull fractures:

Basal skull fractures can be missed on routine x-rays. They may cause CSF leakage through the nose or ears. If suspected, a CT scan with bone windows and neurosurgical consultation is required.

(c) Comminuted and deep skull fractures:

Comminuted skull fractures may require surgical debridement.

6. Posttraumatic Seizures

Give lorazepam 2–4 mg or diazepam 5–10 mg stat, then phenytoin 20 mg/kg load I.V. then phenytoin 100 mg I.V. or P.O. (adjust to weight) every 8 h. Five percent of patients may develop posttraumatic epilepsy.

(a) *Immediate*: Seizures occur within 24 h of injury – negligible predisposition to later seizures.
(b) *Early*: Seizures occur within 1 week of injury – increased risk of later seizures.
(c) *Late*: Seizures occur after the first week of injury – further increased risk of later seizures (epilepsy) [5].

7. Concussion

If patient had a concussion, the head CT scan and neurological examination is normal, and the Glasgow Coma Score is 15, they may be discharged home with a warning to come back if there is any decline in level of consciousness, confusion, focal deficit, vomiting, headache, or seizure.

Patients may have had a transient loss of consciousness at the time of head impact which may be associated with a brief period of amnesia following the head injury. Activities with a risk of head injury should be avoided for 1 week following a concussion if loss of consciousness was less than 1 min and for 2 weeks if loss of consciousness was a few minutes in duration.

8. Normal CT Scan, Abnormal Examination

If the CT scan of the head is normal but the patient has a decreased level of consciousness, confusion, focal deficit, or alcohol or drug intoxication, the patient is admitted to ICU and management is directed to treatable causes. An MRI may help reveal diffuse axonal injury.

References

1. Posner JB, Saper CB, Schiff N, Plum F. Plum and Posner's diagnosis of stupor and coma. 4th ed. New York: Oxford University Press; 2007.
2. Bullock MR, Chesnut R, Ghajar J, Gordon D, Hartl R, Newell DW. Surgical management of acute epidural hematomas. Neurosurgery. 2006;58(3 Suppl):S7–15.
3. Brain Trauma Foundation, AANS, Joint Section of Neurotrauma and Critical Care. Guidelines for the management of severe head injury. J Neurotrauma. 1996;13(11):641–734.
4. Bullock MR, Chesnut R, Ghajar J, Gordon D, Hartl R, Newell DW, Servadei F, Walters BC, Wilberger JE, Surgical Management of Traumatic Brain Injury Author Group. Surgical management of acute subdural hematomas. Neurosurgery. 2006;58(3 Suppl): S16–24.
5. Englander J, Bushnik T, Duong TT, Cifu DX, Zafonte R, Wright J, Hughes R, Bergman W. Analyzing risk factors for late post-traumatic seizures: a prospective, multicenter investigation. Arch Phys Med Rehabil. 2003;84(3):365–73.

Chapter 9
Meningitis and Encephalitis

1. *Meningitis* is characterized by severe generalized headache, fever, neck stiffness and a change in mental status. There is often also nausea, vomiting, photophobia and skin rash. Elderly patients may have minimal symptoms and no fever; change in mental status may be the only feature.
2. *Encephalitis* is characterized by a change in the level of consciousness, seizures, flu-like illness, memory loss, and behavioral changes, with or without fever. Immunosuppressant medications make patients especially susceptible to central nervous system infections.

    Superior longitudinal sinus thrombosis and retropharyngeal abscess (particularly in children) may be mistaken for meningitis because symptoms and signs include severe headache, fever, and resistance to neck flexion.

Stabilize the Patient

ABCs

1. Assess the airway and breathing rate, and look for signs of respiratory distress. If there is respiratory distress or a decreased level of consciousness (especially GCS less than or equal to 8), intubation and ventilation are required.
2. Check the vital signs and assess if the patient is hemodynamically stable. Place the patient on a cardiac monitor and pulse oximeter. Give I.V. fluids.

A.Q. Rana, J.A. Morren, *Neurological Emergencies in Clinical Practice,* DOI 10.1007/978-1-4471-5191-3_9, © Springer-Verlag London 2013

Focused History

Take a focused history of the presenting symptom and onset.

Focused Exam

1. Do a focused neurological examination (see Glasgow Coma Scale, Chap. 1). Include mental status assessment, observation of breathing pattern, pupil size and response, any eye deviation, lateralizing signs, deep tendon reflexes, and plantar responses.
2. Check for meningeal signs (see section "Identify the Underlying Cause"). Look for pertinent skin lesions like non-blanching rash (purpura/petechiae).

STAT Labs and Treatments

1. Start an I.V. line of normal saline.
2. Send blood work: CBC, hematocrit, electrolytes, glucose, creatinine, PT, and INR. Check arterial blood gases and send blood for culture and sensitivity panel. Serum virology may also be needed.
3. Get an ECG, chest x-ray, and urine analysis.
4. Do a STAT CT scan of the head. Consider giving empiric broad-spectrum antibiotics (see section "Treat the Underlying Cause") prior to sending the patient to the scanner.
5. Make arrangements for lumbar puncture after the CT scan of head, including review of PT, INR, and platelet count and getting consent for the procedure. *Do not delay antibiotic treatment of suspected meningitis pending the arrangements for lumbar puncture.*

Identify the Underlying Cause

Take Further History

1. Ask about the duration of symptoms, including neck or back pain, fever, cough, nausea, vomiting, photophobia, shortness of breath, and chest pain.

2. Get a history of immune status and medication use such as chemotherapy/immunosupressants and prednisone.
3. Ask about any recent travel or exposures.
4. Ask about recent ear, nose, throat, and sinus infections and any head and neck surgery or trauma.

Do Further Examination

A complete neurological examination should be done. This includes testing mental status, cranial nerves, muscle bulk, tone, power, adventitious movements, deep tendon reflexes, plantar responses, coordination with station and gait assessment, as well as sensory examination of all modalities.

1. Check for neck stiffness and meningeal signs.

   Brudzinski's sign is present if passive flexion of the patient's neck by the examiner results in flexion of the lower extremities (Fig. 9.1a).

   Kernig's sign is present if, with hip and knee in flexion, passive extension of the knee is restricted by hamstring spasm and/or pain (Fig. 9.1b).

   Meningeal signs have low sensitivity and specificity. Neck stiffness with extension and flexion but normal rotation is a more reliable sign of meningitis. Also, meningismus is not specific to infection, but can be seen in subarachnoid hemorrhage.

2. Examine the fundus for papilledema, and palpate for sinus tenderness.
3. Auscultate lungs and heart to rule out a systemic source of infection. (Patients with meningitis may have systemic sepsis.)
4. Check for petechial rash or palpable purpura, which suggests meningococcal meningitis.

Do Further Investigations

1. CT Scan of Head
   A CT scan of the head is done before lumbar puncture to rule out mass lesion which, if present, may lead to herniation with lumbar puncture.

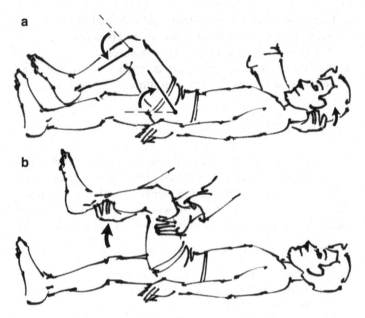

FIGURE 9.1 (a) Brudzinski's sign (b) Kernig's sign

Meningitis: may be normal or show diffuse edema
Encephalitis: may show diffuse or focal edema. If herpetic, may show small necrotizing or hemorrhagic lesions on the inferior frontal and temporal lobes

2. Lumbar Puncture
Send CSF for culture and sensitivity +/– fungal and Gram stains also. For herpes encephalitis, PCR is more reliable than viral cultures but still takes time to get results. CSF may be normal early in herpes encephalitis. Typical CSF findings in various meningitis types are shown in Table 9.1.

3. EEG
The EEG shows characteristic PLEDS (periodic lateralizing epileptiform discharges) in herpes encephalitis.

4. MRI
MRI is more sensitive than CT for detecting the inferior frontal and temporal focal necrotizing lesions of herpes encephalitis.

TABLE 9.1 Typical CSF findings in various meningitis types [1]

CSF	CSF color	WBCs (/mm³)	Protein (mg/dl)	Glucose (mg/dl)	Opening pressure (mmH₂O)
Normal	Clear	<5 (lymphocytic)	15–45	50–85 (2/3 of serum)	80–180
Bacterial meningitis	Cloudy	5–10,000 (PMNs)	Increased	Decreased	Typically increased
Viral meningitis (non-herpetic)	Clear to cloudy	5–1,000 (lymphocytic)	Increased	Normal	Typically normal
Herpes meningoencephalitis	Typically blood tinged	5–200 (lymphocytic) increased RBCs	Increased	Normal	May be increased
Fungal meningitis	Clear to cloudy	Variable count (lymphocytic)	Increased	Decreased	May be increased
Tubercular meningitis	Cloudy	Variable count (lymphocytic)	Increased	Decreased	May be increased

Treat the Underlying Cause

1. Meningitis

   (a) Ceftriaxone 2 g I.V. every 12 h.
   (b) Add ampicillin 1–2 g I.V. every 3–4 h if *Listeria* is suspected (in patients less than 3 months and older than 50 years of age) [2].
   (c) Add vancomycin 1 g every 12 h if *Staphylococcus* is suspected (or *Streptococcus pneumoniae* is suspected in Ontario, Canada, since resistance rate is over 20 %), pending the results of CSF cultures.
   (d) *Use dexamethasone which may decrease morbidity and mortality:*
       With or shortly (10–20 min) before the first dose of antibiotic in all non-immunosuppressed and previously well adults with (suspected or confirmed) pneumococcal meningitis at a dose of 10 mg every 6 h for 4 days and children at a dose of 0.15 mg/kg every 6 h for 4 days for (suspected or confirmed) Haemophilus influenzae type b and pneumococcal meningitis [3].

2. Encephalitis (Viral/Herpetic)

   (a) Acyclovir 10 mg/kg I.V. every 8 h × 10 days.
   (b) Steroids are usually avoided but might be beneficial in some cases [4].

Discussion

Agents Causing Meningitis

1. *Young and Middle-Aged Adults*

   (a) *Streptococcus pneumoniae*
   (b) *Neisseria meningitidis*
   (c) Can be *Haemophilus influenzae* (due to increased immigration and inconsistent vaccinations)

2. *Older Adults*
   More have *Haemophilus influenzae*
3. *Post-neurosurgical Procedure and Head Trauma*

   (a) *Staphylococcus aureus.*
   (b) Gram-negative rods.
   (c) *Streptococcus pneumoniae.*
   (d) *Pseudomonas* may be the cause in post-neurosurgery cases (especially diabetics).

4. *Older Adults with Debilitating Medical Conditions and Alcoholism*

   (a) *Streptococcus pneumoniae*
   (b) Gram-negative rods
   (c) *Haemophilus influenzae*

Agents Causing Encephalitis

1. *Adults*
   Herpes virus type I
2. *Neonates*
   Herpes virus type II
3. *Other Viruses Causing Encephalitis*

   (a) Enteroviruses.
   (b) Echovirus.
   (c) Coxsackievirus.
   (d) Epstein-Barr virus (EBV).
   (e) Cytomegalovirus (CMV).
   (f) West Nile virus should be considered in the fall season.

Meningitis (Meningococcal) Prophylaxis

Rifampin 10–20 mg/kg up to 600 mg twice daily is given to contacts for 2 days.

References

1. Seehusen DA, Reeves MM, Fomin DA. Cerebrospinal fluid analysis. Am Fam Physician. 2003;68(6):1103–8.
2. El Bashir H, Laundy M, Booy R. Diagnosis and treatment of bacterial meningitis. Arch Dis Child. 2003;88(7):615–20.
3. Chaudhuri A, Martinez-Martin P, Kennedy PG, Andrew Seaton R, Portegies P, Bojar M, Steiner I, EFNS Task Force. EFNS guideline on the management of community-acquired bacterial meningitis: report of an EFNS Task Force on acute bacterial meningitis in older children and adults. Eur J Neurol. 2008;15(7): 649–59.
4. Fitch MT, van de Beek D. Drug insight: steroids in CNS infectious diseases – new indications for an old therapy. Nat Clin Pract Neurol. 2008;4(2):97–104.

Chapter 10
Multiple Sclerosis (Exacerbation)

Approximately 85 % of patients with multiple sclerosis (MS) present with the relapsing-remitting form the disease [1]. A high frequency of relapses in the first year after diagnosis is associated with poor prognosis. Treatment of MS exacerbations is the main focus of this chapter.

Stabilize the Patient

ABCs

1. Assess the airway and breathing rate, and look for signs of respiratory distress. Most patients are usually stable.
2. Check the vital signs and assess if the patient is hemodynamically stable. Place the patient on a cardiac monitor and pulse oximeter.

Focused History

1. Take a focused history of the presenting symptoms and onset. Ask the patient for the date of first onset of symptoms of MS and the subsequent date of diagnosis. Ask about how many exacerbations the patients had, how were they treated, and when was the last exacerbation.
2. Exacerbations of multiple sclerosis are characterized by episodes of focal neurological disturbance lasting more

A.Q. Rana, J.A. Morren, *Neurological Emergencies in Clinical Practice,* DOI 10.1007/978-1-4471-5191-3_10, © Springer-Verlag London 2013

than 24 h and preceded by a period of clinical stability lasting 30 days or more [2]. Fluctuations in symptoms with fever, heat, or infection may not be considered true exacerbations since in these contexts previous deficits may be simply "unmasked."

Identify the Underlying Cause

Take Further History

1. Each episode may incompletely resolve leaving the patient with a baseline level of disability. As such, it is important to establish the patient's baseline level of functioning prior to the current relapse to assess the deficits that are actually new.
2. Ask about the history of any precipitating factors and history of disease-modifying therapy (and compliance with treatment) and ask about their regular neurologist and follow-up visit history.

Do Examination

1. A complete neurological examination should be done. This includes testing mental status, cranial nerves, muscle bulk, tone, power, adventitious movements, deep tendon reflexes, plantar responses, coordination with station and gait assessment, as well as sensory examination of all modalities.

Investigations

1. MRI brain with gadolinium may be required in order to assess for any new lesions (usually enhancing) which may be responsible for current exacerbation.
2. CSF is abnormal in the majority of patients. Usually WBC is less than 20 lymphocytes, rarely patients may have up to 50–100. There may be an increase in total protein up to

60 mg/dl; rarely, protein may be elevated up to 100 mg/dl. Myelin basic protein is high in the first couple of weeks of exacerbation, and CSF oligoclonal bands are elevated in majority of patients. IgG synthesis rate and IgG index are usually increased and may be the initial abnormality seen on CSF examination.

3. Visual evoked potentials remain abnormal years after an episode of optic neuritis. Somatosensory and brainstem auditory evoked potentials are abnormal in at least one-third to one-half of patients with MS [3].

Treat the Underlying Cause

Because of the relapsing-remitting nature of the disease and individual variation in therapeutic response, management and treatment of the disease can be very challenging.

1. The commonly used pharmacological agent for acute exacerbations includes corticosteroids. A short course of high-dose methylprednisolone (1 g I.V. per day for 3–7 days) can help to reduce the duration and severity of exacerbations but does not change their frequency. It is usually followed by a tapering course of oral steroids (e.g., prednisone 60–100 mg/day tapered over 4–8 weeks gradually). Blood glucose should be followed closely. GI prophylaxis with H2 blockers or proton pump inhibitors should also be used. Patients should also be monitored for signs and symptoms of infection. Urine analysis, culture, and sensitivity should also be checked.

2. Once the patient is stable, they may be discharged, and decisions regarding disease-modifying therapy can be made in MS clinic or by their regular neurologist. Multiple double-blind multicenter studies have demonstrated that these agents decrease the number and severity of exacerbations in relapsing-remitting MS.

3. The following disease-modifying agents can be used:

Injectables:

Interferon beta-1b (Betaseron®) 0.25 mg SC every other day. Injection sites can be rotated between anterior thigh, buttocks, and abdomen. Patients may be premedicated with ibuprofen, and CBC and LFT should be followed every 3 months. Side effects include injection site reaction, flu-like symptoms, fatigue, drop in WBC, abnormalities in LFTs, and depression.

Interferon beta-1a (Avonex®) 30 µg IM once a week. Side effects include injection site reaction, flu-like symptoms, fever, chills, HA, depression, anxiety, and fatigue. CBC and comprehensive metabolic profile should be followed every 3–6 months.

Interferon beta-1a (Rebif®) 44 µg SC injection three times a week. CBC and LFT should be followed every 3 months. Side effects include injection site reaction, flu-like symptoms, depression, and fatigue.

Glatiramer acetate (Copaxone®) 20 mg SC daily. Side effects include injection site reaction, anxiety, joint pain, transient chest discomfort, and fatigue.

Natalizumab (Tysabri®) 300 mg I.V. once a month (for refractory MS cases). Side effects include infusion reactions, PML, and infections

Oral agents:

Fingolimod (Gilenya®) 0.5 mg P.O. daily. Side effects include headache, transaminitis, diarrhea, bradycardia (severe degree possible with QT prolongation, AV block), and also macular edema. Requires at minimum, ECG at baseline then X6h after first dose and if treatment interrupted. Ophthalmoscopic exams at baseline then 3–4 months after treatment is started. VZV antibody testing at baseline if no past infection or vaccination history.

Teriflunomide (Aubagio®) has been newly approved in the USA and may be considered as an alternative oral option.

Discussion

Exacerbations of MS may be due to known precipitants. Thus, patients need to be treated for such causes concurrently. Some of the common causes include pneumonia, urinary tract and other infections, as well as increases in body temperature which can severely affect nerve conduction through partially demyelinated fibers.

References

1. Goldberg LD, Edwards NC, Fincher C, Doan QV, Al-Sabbagh A, Meletiche DM. Comparing the cost-effectiveness of disease-modifying drugs for the first-line treatment of relapsing-remitting multiple sclerosis. J Manag Care Pharm. 2009;15(7):543–55.
2. Ontaneda D, Rae-Grant AD. Management of acute exacerbations in multiple sclerosis. Ann Indian Acad Neurol. 2009;12(4):264–72.
3. Ko KF. The role of evoked potential and MR imaging in assessing multiple sclerosis: a comparative study. Singapore Med J. 2010;51(9):716–20.

Chapter 11
Myasthenia Gravis

Myasthenia Gravis is characterized by impairment of neuro-muscular junction transmission due to antibody-mediated attack on (mostly) acetylcholine receptors at the postsynaptic membrane. It is associated with the following symptoms and signs:

1. Fluctuating weakness.
2. Excessive fatigability with exercise.
3. Ocular and bulbar muscle involvement, manifesting as ptosis and diplopia, dysarthria, dysphagia, and dyspnea.
4. Limb weakness; proximal muscles are often affected more than distal muscles.

Patients with myasthenia gravis may present to the ER with respiratory failure constituting a myasthenic crisis. This is usually precipitated by infection, surgery, pregnancy, systemic illness, medications, or emotional stress. *It is very important to determine the need for intubation and mechanical ventilation in a timely fashion.* Mortality in myasthenic crisis is about 5 % [1].

Stabilize the Patient

ABCs

1. Assess the airway and breathing rate, and look for signs of respiratory distress.
   Signs of impending respiratory failure:

   (a) Labored or shallow breathing
   (b) Difficulty completing sentences while talking

A.Q. Rana, J.A. Morren, *Neurological Emergencies in Clinical Practice,* DOI 10.1007/978-1-4471-5191-3_11, © Springer-Verlag London 2013

    (c) Use of accessory muscles of respiration
    (d) Inward movements of the abdomen on inspiration (paradoxical respiration)
    (e) A drop in vital capacity (normally 60–70 ml/kg)
    (f) A drop in peak inspiratory pressure (normally greater than –50 cmH$_2$O)

Patients with respiratory compromise may need to be intubated and ventilated irrespective of the arterial blood gases.

2. Dysphagia, often accompanied by a wet gargled voice or poor control of oropharyngeal secretions, is an indication of bulbar muscle weakness and risk of aspiration. Order the patient to be NPO.
3. Check the vital signs and assess if the patient is hemodynamically stable. Place the patient on a cardiac monitor and pulse oximeter.

Focused History

Take a focused history of the presenting symptom and onset, including symptoms of double vision, ptosis, and speech, swallowing, or breathing problems.

Focused Exam

Do a brief neurological exam, focusing on signs of bulbar and respiratory weakness. Suspect neuromuscular respiratory compromise if the patient cannot count up to 20 on a single exhaled breath.

STAT Labs and Treatments

1. Start an I.V. line of normal saline.
2. Send blood work: CBC, electrolytes, glucose, creatinine, PT, and INR. Check arterial blood gases.
3. Get an ECG, chest x-ray, and urine analysis.

Identify the Underlying Cause

Take Further History

1. Ask when myasthenia gravis was diagnosed and how the course has been.
2. Ask about current medications and what medications have been tried in the past
3. Ask about any history of myasthenic crisis, intubations, or admissions in the past.
4. Ask about the onset and duration of the current crisis, and any antecedent infections, stressors, or surgery.

Do Further Examination

A complete neurological examination should be done. This includes testing mental status, cranial nerves, muscle bulk, tone, power, adventitious movements, deep tendon reflexes, plantar responses, coordination with station and gait assessment, as well as sensory examination of all modalities.

1. On cranial nerve examination, look for extraocular muscle weakness and ptosis, with fatigability on prolonged sustained upgaze. There may be facial weakness, and speech may be nasal or "mushy."
2. Screen for fatiguable proximal muscle weakness by repeat motor testing.
3. Auscultate lungs and heart.

Do Further Investigations

Measure vital capacity and peak inspiratory and peak expiratory pressures.

Treat the Underlying Cause

1. Respiratory muscle weakness.
   Early intubation is very important and leads to earlier extubation and a better prognosis. Intubation should not be

guided by arterial blood gases, which are often normal until severe distress occurs. Vital capacity (VC) should be measured at least every 4–6 h if the patient is not intubated and every 12 h if intubated. Do not use noninvasive ventilation (e.g., bilevel positive airway pressure, or BiPAP) if bulbar dysfunction is present since there is increased risk of aspiration.

Guidelines for intubation are:

(a) Clinical signs of respiratory compromise (e.g. tachypnea, use of accessory muscles)
(b) Significant bulbar weakness (e.g. dysphagia with drooling, wet speech); unable to protect airway
(c) Vital capacity drops to 20 ml/kg or less
(d) Maximum expiratory pressure less than 40 cmH_2O and maximum inspiratory pressure weaker than -30 cmH_2O
(e) Blood gases: $pO_2 < 70$, $pCO_2 > 50$, and $pH < 7.35$

Guidelines for ventilation are:

(a) SIMV mode at 8–10 breaths per minute
(b) Tidal volume of 10–15 ml/kg
(c) Positive end expiratory pressure of 5–15 cmH_2O

2. To reduce aspiration risk, the head of the bed should be elevated, chest physiotherapy should be done regularly, and patients should be on NPO.
3. Stop all contraindicated medications. These include aminoglycosides (e.g. gentamicin, streptomycin), tetracycline, doxycycline, clindamycin, azithromycin, ciprofloxacin (and other fluoroquinolones), lithium, thyroxine, procyclidine, lidocaine, penicillamine, chlorpromazine, quinidine, procainamide, and beta blockers such as propranolol or atenolol.
4. In myasthenic crisis, stop acetylcholinesterase inhibitors (e.g., pyridostigmine) as they can cause increased secretions. They may be gently restarted shortly before extubation.
5. Immune-modulating therapy (given after stabilization of patient, including airway protection)

Plasma exchange: This is usually performed on alternate days for a total of five treatments (250 ml of plasma/kg total or removal of 1–1.5 times plasma volume on each session). Side effects include infections, arrhythmias, hypotension, bleeding, and hypocalcemia.

Intravenous immunoglobulin (IVIG): The dose is 0.4 g/kg/ day for 5 days. IVIG reduces the time to recovery and decreases the need for mechanical ventilation. *IgA levels should be checked in all patients* before starting IVIG because of the increased risk of anaphylaxis in patients with IgA deficiency. Side effects of IVIG include headache, renal failure, allergic reactions, aseptic meningitis, hemolytic anemia, and hypercoagulability-related complications like DVT and stroke.

High-dose corticosteroids: prednisone 1 mg/kg/day

Discussion

Investigations in Patients with Newly Diagnosed Myasthenia Gravis

1. Ice pack test.
   Application of covered ice to the eyes for 2–5 min. If positive, there is an appreciable improvement of the patient's ptosis [2].
2. Serological investigations: These include anti-acetylcholine receptor antibodies: AChR-Abs binding, blocking, and modulating. These will be present in up to 80–85 %. In 50 % of the remaining seronegative group, muscle-specific tyrosine kinase (MuSK) antibodies will be positive.
3. Repetitive nerve stimulation test:
   Repetitive nerve stimulation should show a decremental response to low-frequency stimulation (2–5 Hz).
4. Single-fiber EMG:
   Perform this in clinically suspected cases where the repetitive nerve stimulation test is negative.

5. Tensilon test: If an undiagnosed patient presents with crisis symptoms and ptosis, this test may be done to help support a preliminary diagnosis before the results of more definitive testing is available.

   The test is done in a monitored setting with a crash/code cart at the bedside. The patient should have an I.V. line. Note the extent of ptosis present before beginning the test. Then give 2 mg of edrophonium I.V., watching for side effects of hypotension and bradycardia. If no side effects are noticed, inject the remaining 8 mg of edrophonium and watch for improvement of the ptosis. If the patient develops bradycardia, give 0.5–1 mg atropine I.V.

6. CT scan of the chest for detection of thymoma.

7. Other blood work: thyroid function tests, ANA, RF, ESR, CBC, and electrolytes.

Treatments in Patients with Newly Diagnosed Myasthenia Gravis

1. Acetylcholinesterase inhibitors

   Patients who are not in crises and have mild symptoms may be treated only with acetylcholinesterase inhibitors such as pyridostigmine (Mestinon®). Start at a dose of 30–60 mg every 6 h and titrate to a maximum dose of 120 mg every 3 h.

2. Other immunosuppressants

   In more symptomatic individuals who are not likely to be adequately controlled on pyridostigmine alone, use prednisone +/− steroid-sparing agent like azathioprine, mycophenolate mofetil or cyclosporine.

3. Thymectomy

   This is indicated for all patients with thymoma and recommended for patients with severe generalized myasthenia without thymoma (especially if the patient is less than 50 years) [3]. It leads to improvement in about 40 % of patients and remission in about 40 % of patients [4].

Cholinergic Versus Myasthenic Crises

Cholinergic crisis is caused by overmedication and is characterized by increased salivation and secretions, diarrhea, abdominal cramps, miosis, fasciculations, and bradycardia. *Cholinergic crisis must be carefully distinguished from myasthenic crisis because the respective treatments are fundamentally different.* Cholinergic crisis is treated by decreasing the dose of acetylcholinesterase inhibitor medication.

References

1. Thomas CE, Mayer SA, Gungor Y, Swarup R, Webster EA, Chang I, Brannagan TH, Fink ME, Rowland LP. Myasthenic crisis: clinical features, mortality, complications, and risk factors for prolonged intubation. Neurology. 1997;48(5):1253–60.
2. Kearsey C, Fernando P, D'Costa D, Ferdinand P. The use of the ice pack test in myasthenia gravis. JRSM Short Rep. 2010;1(1):14.
3. Gronseth GS, Barohn RJ. Practice parameter: thymectomy for autoimmune myasthenia gravis (an evidence-based review): report of the Quality Standards Subcommittee of the American Academy of Neurology. Neurology. 2000;55(1):7–15.
4. Glinjongol C, Paiboonpol S. Outcome after transsternal radical thymectomy for myasthenia gravis: 14-year review at Ratchaburi Hospital. J Med Assoc Thai. 2004;87(11):1304–10.

Chapter 12
Neck and Back Pain

Acute back and neck pain is a common complaint seen in the emergency department. Chronic pain, lasting more than several months, can be indicative of an underlying back condition such as disk (nucleus pulposus) herniation, spinal stenosis, or cervical spondylosis in cases of neck pain. A comprehensive back or neck pain assessment is required for appropriate treatment [1].

Stabilize the Patient

ABCs

1. Assess the airway and breathing rate, and look for signs of respiratory distress. Patients are usually stable. Trauma patients with acute neck pain should have neck immobilization and x-rays to rule out C-spine instability before moving the neck.
2. Check the vital signs and assess if the patient is hemodynamically stable. Place the patient on a cardiac monitor and pulse oximeter.

Focused History

1. Ask questions about the pain's site, onset, nature, radiation, severity, aggravating/alleviating factors, related injuries,

falls, or trauma. (For neck pain, also ask if they have any swelling or lumps in their neck.)

Focused Exam

1. Inspection of the site of pain for any wounds, bleeding, or skin breakdown. Range of motion, especially flexion and extension, should be assessed. For back pain, also evaluate for paraspinal tenderness.
2. Observing the behavior and position of the patients may help one to get an impression of the connection between their complaints and the level of disability. Check to see if patient is lying or sitting, rolling around, grimacing, moaning, or keeping the affected body area in a fixed posture. Fever may be suggestive of infection. Acute pain may be accompanied by tachycardia and elevated blood pressure.

Identify the Underlying Cause

Take Further History

1. Ask about any additional symptoms, such as weakness, radicular numbness, or tingling (saddle anesthesia in back pain cases), bowel and bladder control, as well as erectile dysfunction.
2. Ask about any previous history of back or neck pain or surgeries done in these areas.
3. Ask about history of malignancies (which may implicate spine metastases, especially with prostate cancer).

Do Further Examination

1. A complete neurological examination should be done. This includes testing mental status, cranial nerves, muscle bulk, tone, power, adventitious movements, deep tendon

reflexes, plantar responses, coordination with station and gait assessment, as well as sensory examination of all modalities.

2. Specific examinations for individual pain syndromes can be done. However, certain aspects are part of most pain assessments-testing joints for active and passive range of motion, looking for signs of inflammation (swelling, tenderness) and percussion of the spine may be helpful. Straight leg raise test (Lasègue's sign) for low back pain can point toward lumbar nerve root compression. Spurling's maneuver and Lhermitte's sign may be relevant in assessing neck pain related to cervical spondylosis [2].

Do Investigations

Imaging tests can be done to determine a structural cause for the pain. These can include x-ray, CT, and/or MRI. Sometimes the use of flexion and extension views is quite informative regarding spine stability. CBC, ESR, or other investigations directed to determine the presence of infection-associated causes are helpful.

Treat the Underlying Cause

1. Severe acute back and neck pain can be treated with various medications such as NSAIDS and opioids, which may be used as the first line of treatment. They are usually fast acting and dosage can be based upon the intensity of pain and limited by adverse effects. Skeletal muscle relaxants (e.g., cyclobenzaprine, tizanidine, metaxalone) are useful since they often augment the effects of analgesics.

2. Tricyclic antidepressants (TCAs) are useful adjuncts for the treatment of chronic back/neck pain. Regular dosing schedules have been shown to achieve better pain control in chronic pain while also minimizing the anxiety of not knowing when the next back/neck pain exacerbation will

occur. Additionally, formal psychological support may be important in the long-term management of such chronic pain.

3. Other treatments include local or regional anesthetic blocks and spinal steroid injections. Physical therapy is quite useful in the treatment of chronic back/neck pain, often done in conjunction with the pharmacological treatments mentioned above.

4. Surgical decision-making is complex but is usually based on the presence of significant, active neural compromise often demonstrated by imaging and electrodiagnostic studies.

Discussion

Waiting to see if the pain goes away or becomes less intense on its own may be deleterious. Peripherally induced central mechanisms (sensitization) may intensify and prolong patient suffering. Additionally, partial treatment of back and neck pain is also shown to be counterproductive to long-term symptom management.

The evaluation of pain can be accomplished through taking an adequate history and performing a physical examination with or without analgesia. Back pain, having a wide spectrum of causes, may present with various symptoms. The pain can be intermittent, constant, or occurring only in certain positions or when performing certain tasks. Pain can be localized or radiate to other areas and can present as sharp, dull aching, piercing, or burning. Patients with neck pain may have difficulty moving neck from side to side or up and down due to neck stiffness from reactive spasm.

Red flags in the evaluation of neck or back pain include objective weakness with either lower motor neuron signs (radicular or hyperacute myelopathic) or upper motor neuron signs (myelopathic). Sensory loss with a level (myelopathic) or in a dermatomal distribution (radicular) and loss of bowel or bladder control would also prompt emergency neurosurgical evaluation for timely intervention.

References

1. Manusov EG. Evaluation and diagnosis of low back pain. Prim Care. 2012;39(3):471–9.
2. Rubinstein SM, Pool JJ, van Tulder MW, Riphagen II, de Vet HC. A systematic review of the diagnostic accuracy of provocative tests of the neck for diagnosing cervical radiculopathy. Eur Spine J. 2007;16(3):307–19.

Chapter 13
Neuroleptic Malignant Syndrome (NMS)

This is a rare neurological emergency with mortality being as high as 38 % in the past. Early diagnosis and improved management have decreased mortality to less than 10 % at present [1]. The causes include typical neuroleptic medications which are potent dopamine antagonists (e.g., chlorpromazine and haloperidol). Timely assessment and treatment is very important.

Clinical features include:

1. Fever
2. Hypertension and autonomic instability
3. Change in mental status
4. Diffuse muscular rigidity
5. Rhabdomyolysis

Stabilize the Patient

ABCs

1. Assess the airway and breathing rate, and look for signs of respiratory distress. If there is respiratory distress or a decreased level of consciousness where airway protection is compromised, intubation and ventilation are required.
2. Check the vital signs and assess if the patient is hemodynamically stable. Place the patient on a cardiac monitor and pulse oximeter. *Autonomic instability is very common.* Give I.V. fluids.

A.Q. Rana, J.A. Morren, *Neurological Emergencies in Clinical Practice*, DOI 10.1007/978-1-4471-5191-3_13, © Springer-Verlag London 2013

Focused History

Take a focused history of the presenting symptoms and onset. A supplemental source of history is likely needed due to the altered mental status of the patient that is expected.

Identify the Underlying Cause

Take Further History

1. Ask about the use of antipsychotics and any of the other medications associated with NMS (see section "Discussion").
2. Ask about sudden cessation of dopaminergic medications.

Do Examination

1. A complete neurological examination should be done. This includes testing mental status, cranial nerves, muscle bulk, tone, power, adventitious movements, deep tendon reflexes, plantar responses, coordination with station and gait assessment, as well as sensory examination of all modalities.
2. Take particular note of mental status, muscular rigidity, blood pressure, and cardiac rhythm.

Do Investigations

Send blood work: CBC, LFTs, and CK. Obtain urinalysis.

The CK and white cell count is usually elevated. Patients may have myoglobinuria and abnormal liver function tests.

Treat the Underlying Cause

1. Stop the offending agent for which this could be an idiosyncratic reaction.

2. Treat fever with cooling blankets.
3. Give I.V. fluids.
4. Give dantrolene intravenously or orally initiated at 2–3 mg/kg total daily doses every 6–8 h titrated up to a total of 10 mg/kg/day.
5. Give bromocriptine P.O. starting at 2.5 mg three to four times daily titrating up to 10 mg four times daily. Continue for 7–10 days before tapering dose over 3 days.
6. Amantadine may be used as an alternative to bromocriptine. Start with 100 mg orally or via gastric tube titrate as needed to a maximum dose of 200 mg every 12 h.
7. *If NMS occurs in the middle of a surgical procedure, stop the offending medication, and ask surgeons to pause when safe to do so for the aforementioned interventions. The procedure may be resumed if features resolve completely and there is consistent hemodynamic stability.*

Discussion

Common Drugs Associated with Neuroleptic Malignant Syndrome

1. Neuroleptic antipsychotics
2. Metoclopramide
3. Levodopa (withdrawal)
4. Carbamazepine
5. Lithium
6. Cocaine (risk increases in combination with neuroleptics) [2]

References

1. Ahuja N, Cole AJ. Hyperthermia syndromes in psychiatry. Adv Psychiatr Treat. 2009;15(3):181–91.
2. Akpaffiong MJ, Ruiz P. Neuroleptic malignant syndrome: a complication of neuroleptics and cocaine abuse. Psychiatr Q. 1991; 62(4):299–309.

Chapter 14
Postherpetic Neuralgia

Herpes zoster (or "shingles") is a painful dermatomal, vesicular rash due to the reactivation of a latent varicella zoster (chicken pox) virus infection in cranial nerve or spinal dorsal root ganglia.

Lifetime incidence of herpes zoster is estimated to be 10–20 %. Risk is increased in immunocompromised individuals.

Using a definition of postherpetic neuralgia as herpes zoster-associated pain lasting 30 or more days, rates reported are as high as 30 % in individuals younger than 40 years and up to 74 % in those above 60 years [1]. The most commonly affected dermatomes are thoracic, cranial (especially trigeminal), lumbar, and cervical.

Herpes zoster ophthalmicus may occur when the virus infects the ophthalmic branch of the trigeminal nerve in the upper face. The rash appears 1–4 days after a prodrome of fever, malaise, and dysesthesias. Vesicular eruption becomes pustular approximately 3 days after, followed by crusts forming by 7–10 days. Diagnosis is made on the basis of the typical dermatomally delineated rash. Pain and mild sensory loss follow the same dermatomal distribution.

Stabilize the Patient

ABCs

1. Assess the airway and breathing rate, and look for signs of respiratory distress.

A.Q. Rana, J.A. Morren, *Neurological Emergencies in Clinical Practice*, DOI 10.1007/978-1-4471-5191-3_14, © Springer-Verlag London 2013

2. Check the vital signs and assess if the patient is hemodynamically stable. Place the patient on a cardiac monitor
   and pulse oximeter. Most patients will be stable.

Focused History

1. Take a focused history of the presenting symptom, onset, and
   course. Ask patient if they recall having chicken pox infection previously or any past exposures/affected contacts.

Focused Exam

1. Determine the borders of the affected area and any
   changes in the sensation of touch and temperature that
   can be noted within that region.

Identify the Underlying Cause

Take Further History

1. Ask about how the pain is affecting the patient's activities
   of daily life, sleep, and interactions with others. Find out if
   the patient is immunocompromised, and review in detail
   all medications that the patient may have tried for the pain,
   including dosages and any side effects that might have
   resulted from them.

Do Further Examination

1. A complete neurological examination should be done. This
   includes testing mental status, cranial nerves, muscle bulk,
   tone, power, adventitious movements, deep tendon reflexes,
   plantar responses, coordination with station and gait assessment, as well as sensory examination of all modalities.

Investigations

In most cases, herpetic neuralgia can be diagnosed by the history and physical examination, and as such no further investigations are required. When the diagnosis is less clear, serology is often also difficult to interpret, however PCR may be used to detect VZV DNA in skin lesions.

Treat the Underlying Cause

Because of the intense pain experienced by these patients, herpetic neuralgia oftentimes presents for emergency treatment. The primary goal of therapy is to shorten the clinical course, provide analgesia, and reduce the risk of developing postherpetic neuralgia.

1. Acyclovir 800 mg by mouth five times per day for 7 days, starting within 72 h of symptom onset. For immunocompromised patients use 10 mg/kg intravenously three times a day for 7 days. However, Acyclovir has not consistently shown reduction in the incidence or severity of postherpetic neuralgia.
2. Prednisone 60 mg PO daily for 7 days (+/− taper) may reduce the acute pain and could potentially reduce the incidence of postherpetic neuralgia [2]. However, prednisone should not be administered to immunocompromised individuals.
3. The following medications may be tried for pain control:

   • Pregabalin, starting dose 50–75 mg twice daily, gradually increased to 150 mg twice daily with a maximum dose of 300 mg twice daily.
   • Gabapentin starting dose of 100 mg, one to three times daily can be gradually increased to 300 mg three times daily, and maximum dose of 600 mg three times daily can be used. Slower escalation rate is indicated in the elderly.
   • Carbamazepine 100 mg two times a day to 800 mg/day may be another option.

Discussion

Management of postherpetic neuralgia can be a challenge and sometimes requires a combination of the aforementioned analgesic medications. Zoster vaccine (Zostavax®) is now available as an option for the prevention of herpes zoster and associated herpetic neuralgia.

References

1. Yawn BP. Post-shingles neuralgia by any definition is painful, but is it PHN? Mayo Clin Proc. 2011;86(12):1141–2.
2. Stankus SJ, Dlugopolski M, Packer D. Management of herpes zoster (shingles) and postherpetic neuralgia. Am Fam Physician. 2000;61(8):2437–44, 2447–8.

Chapter 15
Pseudotumor Cerebri

Pseudotumor cerebri is also known as benign/idiopathic intracranial hypertension. Patients with pseudotumor cerebri are usually young, obese females, who may have a history of medication use including tetracycline, steroids, or vitamin A and its derivatives.

Symptoms and signs may include:

1. Generalized headache
2. Transient visual obscurations
3. Papilledema
4. Cranial nerve VI palsy (a nonlocalizing sign)

In pregnant or postpartum patients, the differential includes venous sinus thrombosis, which must be ruled out with an MRV.

There is significant risk of permanent loss of vision in untreated patients; therefore, it is practically a medical emergency and should be appropriately considered in the differential diagnosis of headache.

Stabilize the Patient

ABCs

1. Assess the airway and breathing rate, and look for signs of respiratory distress.

A.Q. Rana, J.A. Morren, *Neurological Emergencies in Clinical Practice,* DOI 10.1007/978-1-4471-5191-3_15, © Springer-Verlag London 2013

2. Check the vital signs and assess if the patient is hemodynamically stable. Most patients will be stable.

Focused History

Take a focused history of the presenting symptom and onset.

Identify the Underlying Cause

Take Further History

1. Ask about the onset, frequency, and nature of headaches and transient visual obscurations. Patients describe a dimming of vision which lasts for seconds and which occurs with change in position, especially on standing up.
2. Ask about the use of vitamin A and its derivatives (e.g., retinoids), tetracycline, and steroids.
3. Ask about associated conditions such as pregnancy, other hypercoagulable states, and sinus infections.

Do Examination

1. A complete neurological examination should be done. This includes testing mental status, cranial nerves, muscle bulk, tone, power, adventitious movements, deep tendon reflexes, plantar responses, coordination with station and gait assessment, as well as sensory examination of all modalities.
2. Pay particular attention to papilledema (Fig. 15.1), enlarged blind spot, loss of the inferonasal visual field, generalized constriction of the visual field (in advanced cases), and cranial nerve VI palsy [1, 2].

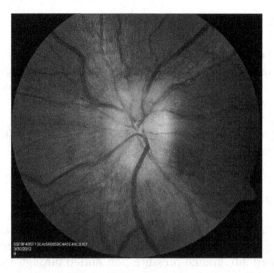

FIGURE 15.1 Grade III papilledema showing blurred disc margins and disc vessels obscuration by the nerve fiber layer. There are very prominent peripapillary nerve fibers (Courtesy of Dr. Lisa Lystad, Cleveland Clinic)

Do Investigations

1. CT/MRI scan of head.

   A CT scan of the head can be normal or show slit-like ventricles.

2. Lumbar puncture.

   The opening pressure is elevated above 250 mm H_2O, but the rest of the CSF analysis should be normal, with possible exception of a low protein level [3].

3. MRV.

   Done to rule out venous sinus thrombosis in pregnant, postpartum, or other high-risk patients.

4. Formal visual field testing is done to screen for and monitor any visual field loss.

Treat the Underlying Cause

1. The offending agent should be stopped.
2. Weight loss is the mainstay of long-term management.
3. Acetazolamide 250 mg three times daily or furosemide 40–80 mg daily may be helpful [4].
4. Patients may need a VP shunt.
5. Optic nerve sheath fenestration is indicated in refractory patients.

Discussion

Untreated intracranial hypertension may result in permanent loss of vision due to compression of the optic nerve by increased intracranial pressure transmitted through the sub-arachnoid space.

References

1. Wall M, Hart Jr WM, Burde RM. Visual field defects in idiopathic intracranial hypertension (pseudotumor cerebri). Am J Ophthalmol. 1983;96(5):654–69.
2. Rowe FJ, Sarkies NJ. Assessment of visual function in idiopathic intracranial hypertension: a prospective study. Eye (Lond). 1998; 12(Pt 1):111–8.
3. Johnston PK, Corbett JJ, Maxner CE. Cerebrospinal fluid protein and opening pressure in idiopathic intracranial hypertension (pseudotumor cerebri). Neurology. 1991;41(7):1040–2.
4. Wall M. Idiopathic intracranial hypertension. Neurol Clin. 2010;28(3):593–617.

Chapter 16
Seizures and Status Epilepticus

Seizures are caused by abnormal excessive synchronous discharges of cortical neurons which produce a sudden change in neurological function. Seizures may be generalized, focal, or focal onset with secondary generalization. Most seizures last many seconds to minutes, but persistent seizure activity (status epilepticus) can also occur.

1. *Generalized seizures* involve both hemispheres of the brain simultaneously, usually cause a decline in level of consciousness, and can be tonic, atonic, clonic, tonic-clonic or nonmotor (e.g., absence seizures).
2. *Focal seizures* are also known as partial seizures and originate from a lateralized focus in the brain.

   (a) *Simple partial seizures*: no impairment in the level of consciousness
   (b) *Complex partial seizures*: impairment in the level of consciousness

3. *Status epilepticus* can be convulsive or nonconvulsive.

   (a) *Convulsive status epilepticus*: variably defined as continuous seizure activity lasting 5–30 min or as two or more serial seizures without return to normal level of consciousness in between episodes (interictally)
   (b) *Nonconvulsive status epilepticus*: Patients may appear confused or aphasic or have profound depressed sensorium. The diagnosis of nonconvulsive status epilepticus is made by a combination of clinical features and EEG findings.

A.Q. Rana, J.A. Morren, *Neurological Emergencies in Clinical Practice,* DOI 10.1007/978-1-4471-5191-3_16, © Springer-Verlag London 2013

Stabilize the Patient

If Actively Seizing

At the Bedside (First 3–5 min)

1. Turn the patient to the lateral decubitus position to prevent aspiration (the "recovery position"). Apply pulse oximeter.
2. Start oxygen by nasal cannula.
3. Turn the side rails of the bed up (rails should be padded).

Focused History and Examination

1. Take a focused history from witnesses or family member if available. Also review EMS/ambulance service record.
2. Note whether the seizure is focal or generalized at onset versus having secondary generalization after a focal onset.
3. Determine the level of consciousness by asking questions such as "close your eyes" or "stick out your tongue" or "tell me your name" or "show me your right hand."

STAT Labs and Treatments

1. Obtain finger-stick glucose. If hypoglycemic, *always give 100 mg of intravenous thiamine* before giving glucose 50 ml of D50W I.V., to prevent Wernicke's encephalopathy.
2. Get STAT blood work for blood glucose, complete blood count, comprehensive metabolic panel, calcium (total and ionized), phosphate and magnesium. Based on clinical presentation may add serial troponins, type and hold, coagulation studies, arterial blood gas, serum alcohol level, toxicology screen (urine and blood), and inborn errors of metabolism screen [1].
3. If the patient is on antiepileptic medications (see Table 16.1), check antiepileptic drug (AED) levels and order an ECG.

Table 16.1 Commonly used antiepileptic medications

Drug	Mechanism	t1/2 (h)	Therapeutic Level
Phenytoin	Na channel modulation	6–30	10–20 µg/ml or 40–80 µmol/L
Carbamazepine	Na channel blocker	12–17	4–12 µg/ml or 17–47 µmol/L
Valproic acid	Multiple: Na channel blocker, GABA potentiation, and glutamate and NMDA inhibition	6–16	50–100 µg/ml or 350–700 µmol/L
Phenobarbital	Enhances GABA inhibition	50–96	15–40 µg/ml or 70–168 µmol/L
Topiramate	(Complex mechanisms) Na channel blocker	18–30	N/A
Lamotrigine	Na channel blocker	24	1–20 µg/ml
Gabapentin	Alpha-2-delta calcium channel subunit blocker	5–8	2–20 µg/ml
Felbamate	Glutamate-glycine blocker (binds to NMDA receptors)	18	30–60 µg/ml
Primidone	GABA agonist sodium channel modulation	6–18	6–12 µg/ml
Ethosuximide	L-type calcium channel blocker	56–60	40–100 µg/ml
Tiagabine	GABA uptake inhibitor	5–8	N/A
Oxcarbazepine	Na channel blocker	8	N/A
Levetiracetam	Synaptic vesicle protein 2A blocker	5–8	N/A
Lacosamide	Sodium channel slow inactivation	13	N/A

If the Seizure Does Not Stop Spontaneously in 3–5 min

1. Assess the respiratory status; get an oral airway and Ambu bag ready.
2. Start two I.V. lines; run 250 ml normal saline to keep the veins open (TKVO).
3. Give:

   Lorazepam 2 mg I.V. at a rate of less than or equal to 2 mg/min (total dose of 0.1 mg/kg) or *diazepam* 5–10 mg I.V. every 5–10 min to a maximum of 30 mg.
   Watch for respiratory depression.

4. If still seizing and there is no history of allergies to phenytoin, give:

   Fosphenytoin 20 mg PE/kg at a rate of less than or equal to 150 mg PE/min.
   If the I.V. site is not available, fosphenytoin can be given I.M., or if fosphenytoin is not available (in many provinces of Canada), give:
   Phenytoin 20 mg/kg at a rate of less than or equal to 50 mg/min.
   Watch for hypotension and cardiac arrhythmia.

If Seizing Continues

Give additional I.V. fosphenytoin (or phenytoin) to a maximum total dose of 30 mg PE/kg, then:

1. Intubate (if not already done).
2. Give one of the following:

   Phenobarbital I.V. load of 15–20 mg/kg at a rate of 75 mg/min OR
   Midazolam I.V. at 0.2 mg/kg, repeat in 5 min then followed by 0.1–2 mg/kg/h OR
   Propofol 1–2 mg/kg load, repeat in 5 min followed by 1–5 mg/kg/h I.V. OR
   Valproic acid 30–40 mg/kg I.V. load followed by 10–15 mg/kg q6h [2] OR

Valproate I.V. 25–30 mg/kg at 3 mg/kg/min OR
Levetiracetam I.V. 20 mg/kg over 15 min

Most Seizures Stop at This Point, But if Seizing Continues

If the patient still does not stop seizing after a benzodiaz-epine and two other anticonvulsants have been given:

1. Give: *Pentobarbital* 5 mg/kg load (<50 mg/min), then 0.5–5 mg/kg/h

   Many hospitals use propofol before trying pentobarbital because of its shorter duration of action.

2. Get a STAT CT scan of the head (before EEG electrodes connection).
3. Continuous EEG monitoring is important; if seizure per-sists, continue I.V. infusion of midazolam, propofol, and pentobarbital and titrate dose to target level of burst sup-pression pattern.
4. Consult anesthesia. General anesthesia may be required if the patient is still refractory.

If No Longer Seizing

Generally, for a single seizure lasting 5 min or less, no acute treatment is necessary.

At the Bedside

1. Turn the patient to the lateral decubitus position to pre-vent aspiration.
2. Turn the padded side rails of the bed up.
3. Check vital signs and level of consciousness every 15 min for 1 h, then every 30 min for 1 h, then every 1 h for 2 h, and then every 4 h.

STAT Labs and Treatments

1. Start an I.V. line; run 250 ml of normal saline to keep veins open.
2. Get blood work for CBC, serum glucose, electrolytes, calcium (total and ionized), phosphate, magnesium, AST, ALT, BUN, creatinine, serum alcohol level, and a urine and serum drug screen.
3. If the patient takes antiepileptic medications, check antiepileptic drug levels.

Identify the Underlying Cause

Take Further History

1. Ask if this is the first seizure or if there is a prior history of seizures.
2. If there is a prior history of seizures:

   (a) Note whether this seizure is similar to previous seizures or not.
   (b) Ask when the last seizure occurred.
   (c) Take a detailed history of the onset, pattern, and frequency of seizures. Include questions about any aura, tongue biting, incontinence, and postictal confusion and whether all the seizures are the same or if they have different types. Get descriptions of witnessed seizures.
   (d) Ask about compliance with medications, any over the counter medications taken, sleep deprivation, unusual stressors and symptoms of intercurrent infection.
   (e) Get details regarding neurologist visits, medications previously used, and details of previous work-up including brain CT, MRI, EEG and epilepsy monitoring unit evaluation.

3. Ask about risk factors for seizures:

   (a) Childhood febrile seizures
   (b) Birth and developmental problems

    (c) Family history of seizures
    (d) Head trauma
    (e) Meningitis or encephalitis
    (f) Alcohol or drug abuse such as cocaine and amphetamine
    (g) Medication use such as theophylline, lidocaine, demerol, tramadol, and bupropion
    (h) Pregnancy and eclampsia

4. Ask about systemic symptoms and general health including a history of:

    (a) Being immunocompromised or diabetic
    (b) Hypoglycemic episodes
    (c) Dementia
    (d) Any fever in the last 24 h
    (e) Sudden severe headache
    (f) Prior episodes of loss of consciousness

5. Ask about neurological symptoms:

    (a) New onset headaches
    (b) Change in personality
    (c) New memory or cognitive dysfunction
    (d) Problems with vision, speech, or swallowing
    (e) Weakness or sensory disturbance
    (f) Bowel or bladder dysfunction

Do Further Examination

1. A complete neurological examination should be done. This includes testing mental status, cranial nerves, muscle bulk, tone, power, adventitious movements, deep tendon reflexes, plantar responses, coordination with station and gait assessment, as well as sensory examination of all modalities.
2. Pay particular attention to fundoscopy, any focal motor or sensory signs, and plantar reflexes.
3. Assess neck stiffness and look for meningeal signs. Conventional meningeal signs have low sensitivity and

specificity. Neck stiffness with extension and flexion, but normal rotation is a more reliable sign of meningitis. Also, meningismus is not specific to infection but can be seen in subarachnoid hemorrhage.

> *Brudzinski's sign* is present if passive flexion of the patient's neck by the examiner results in flexion of the lower extremities (see Fig. 9.1).
>
> *Kernig's sign* is present if, with hip and knee in flexion, passive extension of the knee is restricted by hamstring spasm and/or pain (see Fig. 9.2).

4. Examine skin for stigmata of neurocutaneous disorders – for example, adenoma sebaceum, ash leaf spots, Shagreen patches, café au lait spots, and neurofibromas.

Do Further Investigations

1. CT Scan of the Head
   Do a CT scan to rule out epidural hematoma, subdural hematoma, subarachnoid hemorrhage, intracerebral hemorrhage, stroke, tumor, or other focal lesions such as abscess and those seen in neurocysticercosis.

2. Lumbar Puncture
   Lumbar puncture is done *if the CT head is normal* and if meningitis or encephalitis is suspected. The treatment of these conditions should not be postponed pending arrangements for lumbar puncture; if clinically suspected, empiric treatment should be started (see Chap. 9 for details).

3. MRI with Gadolinium and MRA
   Brain MRI with gadolinium with thin coronal slices through hippocampus (seizure protocol) +/– MRA.

4. EEG
   A routine EEG may be normal. This should be followed by a sleep-deprived EEG or an ambulatory EEG or even epilepsy monitoring unit stay.

Common Causes of Seizures

1. The cause of seizures varies in prevalence with age:

    (a) *Under 30*: idiopathic epilepsy is most common.
    (b) *30–60*: idiopathic epilepsy is still most common, but the risk of intracranial tumors is significantly higher than in younger age groups.
    (c) *Over 60*: cerebrovascular disease, intracranial tumors, idiopathic epilepsy

2. Overall, the important causes of seizures are as follows:

    (a) Idiopathic epilepsy
    (b) Toxic: alcohol and drug (cocaine, amphetamine, PCP) withdrawal or intoxication and medications
    (c) Metabolic: hyponatremia, hypocalcaemia, hypomagnesemia, hypoglycemia, uremia, and ammonia abnormalities
    (d) Infection: herpes simplex encephalitis, meningitis, brain abscess, and neurocysticercosis
    (e) Intracranial focal pathologies: subdural or epidural hematoma, intracerebral or subarachnoid hemorrhage, aneurysms, arteriovenous malformation, stroke, brain tumors and metastases

Treat the Underlying Cause

1. Identify the cause of seizure and treat accordingly.
2. If this is a first seizure, decide if the patient needs antiepileptic medications or should be observed. The risks of seizure recurrence and benefits of antiepileptic medication should be discussed (see below) [3].

First Single Seizure

A new onset single generalized seizure may not need to be treated, especially if it is "provoked"– associated with an acute febrile illness, electrolyte or glucose abnormality, sleep deprivation, alcohol or drug withdrawal or intoxication, or if occurred immediately after trauma.

However, if the EEG or neurological examination is abnormal (focal) or there is a brain tumor, history of stroke or vascular malformation, strong family history of epilepsy, concurrent meningitis or encephalitis, and the patient presented in status epilepticus or had a witnessed focal onset, antiepileptic medications should be considered.

Recurrent Seizures

If there is a previous history of seizures and the patient is already on antiepileptic medications, the drug levels of antiepileptic medications are checked. If the level is subtherapeutic then the dosage of antiepileptic medication is adjusted to the upper therapeutic range or until the patient experiences any side effects. It may take five half lives for the drug level to stabilize in a steady state.

Remember that antiepileptic drug levels are only guidelines. If seizures are not controlled on one antiepileptic medication at its highest therapeutic levels, only then add a second antiepileptic medication possibly with a different mechanism of action. Watch carefully for drug interactions.

Nonconvulsive Status Epilepticus

See section "Stabilize the Patient".

Discussion

Important Issues to Discuss with the Patient

1. Driving
   The ministry of transportation MOT/DMV should be informed (depending upon provincial/state regulations) [4].

2. Other Precautions
   Swimming, bathtub use, operating machines, working on heights, ladders, sports, over the counter medications, efficacy of oral contraceptives, pregnancy, teratogenic and other side effects of antiepileptic medications (like bone density loss), drug and alcohol abuse, sleep deprivation, and other conditions which may lower the seizure threshold should be discussed.

References

1. Brophy GM, Bell R, Claassen J, Alldredge B, Bleck TP, Glauser T, Laroche SM, Riviello Jr JJ, Shutter L, Sperling MR, Treiman DM, Vespa PM, Neurocritical Care Society Status Epilepticus Guideline Writing Committee. Guidelines for the evaluation and management of status epilepticus. Neurocrit Care. 2012;17(1):3–23.
2. Gilad R, Izkovitz N, Dabby R, Rapoport A, Sadeh M, Weller B, Lampl Y. Treatment of status epilepticus and acute repetitive seizures with i.v. valproic acid vs phenytoin. Acta Neurol Scand. 2008;118(5):296–300.
3. Marson AG. When to start antiepileptic drug treatment and with what evidence? Epilepsia. 2008;49 Suppl 9:3–6.
4. Classen S, Crizzle AM, Winter SM, Silver W, Eisenschenk S. Evidence-based review on epilepsy and driving. Epilepsy Behav. 2012;23(2):103–12.

Chapter 17
Spinal Cord Compression

Spinal cord compression is a serious neurological emergency and should be evaluated without delay. The prognosis of spinal cord compression depends on the nature and extent of the injury as well as the timely assessment and initiation of treatment. Patients who are brought to the hospital already paraplegic may not be able to walk again even after treatment. Therefore, actions should be expedient.

Symptoms and signs:

1. Bilateral weakness of the lower extremities +/– both upper extremities
2. Loss of sensation with a sensory level
3. Bowel or bladder involvement (sphincteric dyscontrol), erectile dysfunction.

Stabilize the Patient

ABCs

1. Assess the airway and breathing rate, and look for signs of respiratory distress. Any use of accessory respiratory muscles or shallow, labored breathing is a sign of respiratory distress, and intubation must be performed (without neck movement if cervical cord injury is suspected).

A.Q. Rana, J.A. Morren, *Neurological Emergencies in Clinical Practice,* DOI 10.1007/978-1-4471-5191-3_17, © Springer-Verlag London 2013

Injuries above the C5 level may cause respiratory depression.

2. Check the vital signs and assess if the patient is hemodynamically stable. Place the patient on a cardiac monitor and pulse oximeter. Start I.V. fluids or pressors if required. *Patients with a complete transection of the spinal cord may develop hypotension and bradycardia (neurogenic shock) due to sympathetic dysfunction* and therefore should be closely monitored.

Focused History

Take a focused history of the presenting symptom and the onset. *If there is history of trauma and spinal cord injury is suspected, the spine should be immobilized before proceeding any further.*

Focused Exam

Do a focused neurological exam. Include assessment of muscle tone for spasticity or flaccidity (as can be seen acutely in "spinal shock"), strength in the upper and lower extremities, sensory modalities with sensory level, deep tendon reflexes, plantar responses, anal sphincter tone, reflex penile erections in males, and perineal sensory loss (saddle anesthesia) or sparing [1].

STAT Labs and Treatments

1. Start I.V. fluids.
2. Send blood work: CBC, CMP, PT, and INR. Type blood and hold in case transfusion is required.
3. Call the MRI department to get prepared for spinal cord compression study.
4. Call the neurosurgery (or spine) service regarding a possible spinal cord compression case.

Identify the Underlying Cause

Take Further History

1. Take a detailed history emphasizing onset and duration of symptoms, differential weakness of lower or upper extremities, sensory symptoms involving loss of sensation or numbness, back pain, and bowel or bladder symptoms.
2. Ask about injuries and constitutional symptoms such as fever, chills, history of cancers, intravenous drug abuse, infections, HIV, and immune status.

Do Further Examination

A complete neurological examination should be done. This includes testing mental status, cranial nerves, muscle bulk, tone, power, adventitious movements, deep tendon reflexes, plantar responses, coordination with station and gait assessment, as well as sensory examination of all modalities.

1. Rule out papilledema.
   Increased intracranial pressure can result from a parasagittal mass lesion or falx meningioma which may cause bilateral lower extremity weakness and bowel or bladder symptoms.
2. Check for a sensory level by using a safety pin, starting from the lower extremities.
3. Assess perineal sensation.

   > *Sensory loss* (*saddle anesthesia*): suggest injury to the conus medullaris or cauda equina
   >
   > *Sensory sparing*: suggest an intracord or incomplete cord lesion

4. Assess anal sphincter tone.
   The absence of voluntary contraction of the anal sphincter around the finger indicates involvement of the conus

medullaris or cauda equina. There would also be loss of the bulbocavernosus reflex and the anal wink reflex acutely due to spinal shock [2].

5. Compare reflexes of upper and lower extremities.

> Hyperreflexia in the lower extremities disproportionate to the upper extremities often indicates thoracic cord involvement.
>
> Hyperreflexia in both upper and lower extremities indicates cervical cord (or more rostral) involvement.

6. Babinski's sign may be the earliest indication of spinal cord involvement.

Do Further Investigations

1. MRI with gadolinium is the modality of choice in spinal cord compression.
   Call neurosurgery from the MRI suite, as neurosurgeons generally like to review the MRI with the radiologist.
2. A spine CT scan may be superior in trauma cases: This choice should also be discussed with the spine/ neurosurgeon.

Causes of Spinal Cord Compression

1. Trauma
   Symptoms and signs: develop over minutes to hours, and there is often a history of motor vehicle accident, sports or similar injury.
   Myelopathy may develop more quickly than expected because of other complications such as bleeding, dislocation, and instability of the spine.
2. Neoplasm (Fig. 17.1)
   Symptoms and signs: Weakness, loss of sensation, and bowel or bladder involvement usually develop over days or longer.

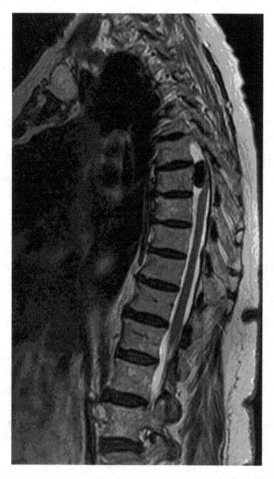

FIGURE. 17.1 MRI showing spinal cord compression at T7 due to a mass lesion

Metastatic tumors often involve the thoracic spine because the venous drainage of many visceral organs is through the spinal extradural venous plexuses (Batson's plexus).

Nerve sheath tumors including meningiomas, neurofibromas, and schwannomas also primarily affect the thoracic region. They arise from spinal roots but cause cord compression on expansion.

Primary neoplasms can be seen at any level.

3. Degenerative Disease of the Spine

   Symptoms and signs: Usually there is a history of radicular neck or back pain.

   This occurs mostly in the cervical region; involvement of thoracic region is very rare. The cervical disks usually herniate centrally, whereas lumbar disks herniate laterally. L1–L2 herniation may cause cauda equina syndrome.

4. Infections

   Symptoms and signs: develop over hours to days, and there may be constitutional symptoms such as fever, chills, night sweats, anorexia, and weight loss.

   Infectious diseases of the spine mostly affect the thoracic and lumbar regions.

   Epidural abscesses caused by bacteria such as *Staphylococcus* may be seen in I.V. drug abusers.

   Vertebral osteomyelitis caused by *Staphylococcus* and *Streptococcus* may cause pathological fractures.

   Spinal tuberculosis (Pott's disease) may be seen in immunocompromised patients or patients with pulmonary TB.

5. Other Causes

   Rheumatoid arthritis may cause atlantoaxial subluxation and rarely epidural and subdural hematomas. Trisomy 21 patients are also at increased risk for atlantoaxial subluxation.

   Arteriovenous malformations of the spine are also rare.

   Congenital anomalies of the spine such as Arnold-Chiari malformation, with or without syringomyelia, may cause myelopathy.

Treat the Underlying Cause

1. Discuss diagnosis and management with the patient and family.
2. Manage spinal cord edema with steroids as follows, include GI protection and blood glucose monitoring.

    (a) For suspected spinal cord tumor:
    Dexamethasone 10 mg I.V. bolus followed by 4 mg every 6 h
    (b) For acute traumatic spinal cord injury (within 8 h following closed spinal cord injury):
    Methylprednisolone 30 mg/kg I.V. bolus over 15 min. After 45 min give methylprednisolone 5.4 mg/kg/h over next 23 h.

3. Surgical treatment is needed in most patients.
    Patients with a tumor may need a biopsy as some tumors may be radiosensitive. Most neoplasms require decompressive laminectomy to relieve pressure on the spinal cord followed by treatment of the primary neoplasm which could be surgery or radiation. Decompressive laminectomy with drainage is needed in most cases of epidural abscess along with I.V. antibiotics. Fractures, dislocation, and subluxation may require open reduction.

References

1. Chapelle PA, Durand J, Lacert P. Penile erection following complete spinal cord injury in man. Br J Urol. 1980;52(3):216–9.
2. Comarr AE. Neurourology of spinal cord-injured patients. Semin Urol. 1992;10(2):74–82.

Chapter 18
Stroke and TIA

Transient ischemic attack (TIA) is defined as a transient episode of neurological dysfunction caused by focal brain, spinal cord, or retinal ischemia, without acute infarction [1]. A stroke occurs with progression to acute infarction in this context.

Patients with ischemic stroke usually present with sudden onset of hemiparesis, facial droop, hemisensory loss, aphasia, dysarthria, hemianopsia, ataxia, diplopia, or vertigo. These patients should be assessed promptly because there is a therapeutic window of 4.5 h after symptom onset for giving intravenous thrombolysis with tissue plasminogen activator (t-PA) [2]. Even within this timeframe, earlier thrombolytic therapy is associated with better functional outcomes. Hemorrhagic stroke typically presents with sudden severe headache, focal weakness, and usually pronounced altered mental status.

Stabilize the Patient

ABCs

1. Assess the airway and breathing rate, and look for signs of respiratory distress. If there is evidence of respiratory distress (especially if GCS is less than or equal to 8), proceed to intubation.

A.Q. Rana, J.A. Morren, *Neurological Emergencies in Clinical Practice*, DOI 10.1007/978-1-4471-5191-3_18, © Springer-Verlag London 2013

2. Check the vital signs and assess if the patient is hemodynamically stable. Place the patient on a cardiac monitor and pulse oximeter. Start I.V. fluids. Avoid dextrose-containing/hypotonic fluids.
3. Monitor vital signs continuously and do not treat hypertension unless above 220/120 mmHg. *Aggressive lowering of blood pressure may precipitate or extend cerebral infarction.*

Focused History

1. Take a focused history of the presenting symptom and the onset. *Ask about the exact time of onset of symptoms.* If the time of onset of symptoms is not clear or if the patient woke up with symptoms from sleep, find out when the patient was last seen in a normal state. That is considered the time of onset for the purposes of I.V. thrombolysis.
2. Determine if the symptoms have resolved, are improving, worsening, or persistent.
3. Ask questions to rule out seizure or bleed (acute onset of sudden severe headache).
4. Determine if the patient is on warfarin or on any antiplatelet medications.

Focused Exam

Perform the NIH stroke scale. Do a focused neurological examination. Include assessment of aphasia, hemianopia, pupils, facial asymmetry, and focal motor and sensory signs, including extinction, inattention/neglect, and plantar reflexes.

STAT Labs and Treatments (Done Simultaneously with Focused History and Exam)

1. Start I.V. fluids with normal saline. *Avoid any hypotonic fluids which may aggravate cerebral edema.*
2. Send STAT blood work: CBC, electrolytes, glucose, creatinine, PT, and INR.

3. Get an ECG.
4. Call the radiology suite to get prepared for a STAT brain CT scan/CT angiogram +/– brain CT perfusion scan, and stroke protocol MRI brain scan. Accompany patient to radiology suite to provide history and tentative localization to the radiologist.
5. Update the I.V. thrombolysis team of a possible case for I.V. t-PA.

Identify the Underlying Cause

Take Further History

1. Get further details of the history regarding the evolution of current symptoms.
2. Inquire about risk factors of stroke including:

   Hypertension, diabetes, hypercholesterolemia, coronary artery disease or cardiac arrhythmias, family history of stroke, prior stroke or TIA, smoking and alcohol.

3. Ask about current medications.

Do Further Examination

1. A complete neurological examination should be done. This includes testing mental status, cranial nerves, muscle bulk, tone, power, adventitious movements, deep tendon reflexes, plantar responses, coordination with station and gait assessment, as well as sensory examination of all modalities.

Do Further Investigations

Review the head CT scan/CT angiogram +/– head CT perfusion scan and stroke protocol MRI brain scan with the radiologist:

1. Rule out hemorrhage.
2. Look for early signs of ischemic infarct especially in areas corresponding to anatomic localization based on deficit [3]:

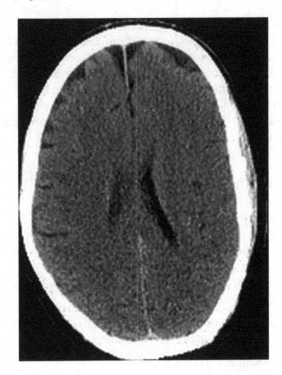

FIGURE 18.1 Non-contrasted head CT scan showing sulcal efface-ment: an early sign of acute (left middle cerebral artery) ischemic infarct (Courtesy of Dr. L. Georgevitch)

Hyperdense MCA sign, sulcal effacement (Fig. 18.1), obscuration of lenticular nucleus, loss of gray-white demar-cation, and insular ribbon sign.

These early signs are subtle compared to those seen later on CT (Fig. 18.2).

t-PA is usually withheld if infarct volume estimated by early changes on CT or MRI is more than 1/3 the MCA ter-ritory especially if between 3 and 4.5 h since symptom onset.

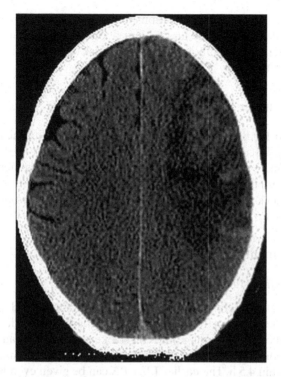

FIGURE 18.2 Non-contrasted head CT scan showing acute ischemic infarct in left middle cerebral artery distribution (Courtesy of Dr. M. Prieditis)

Treat the Underlying Cause

CT Scan Normal or Early Signs of Ischemic Infarct and Patient Is Candidate for t-PA

1. If the patient's symptoms are persistent and significant, the onset was less than 4.5 h ago, and there is no history of seizure activity and no suspicion of intracerebral or subarachnoid hemorrhage, call the I.V. thrombolysis team. *Note: Intra-arterial t-PA may be used in some centers but only in carefully selected patients who have missed the 4.5-h window.*

2. Screen for contraindications to thrombolysis (see below).
3. Talk to the family and patient about indications and side effects of thrombolysis including a risk of hemorrhage with I.V. t-PA.

Do Further Examination after NIH Stroke Scale

1. Do further neurological exam, as time permits, including fundoscopy, full cranial nerve, cerebellar, and tone evaluation, and detailed sensory exam including assessment for hemineglect, astereognosis, and agraphesthesia.
2. Check the pulse, and listen for carotid and ocular/ophthalmic bruits and cardiac murmurs.

Treatment with Intravenous t-PA

Indications for I.V. t-PA:

1. Acute ischemic stroke with significant deficit, NIH stroke scale score of four or more, *or* a particularly eloquent deficit (like language) if NIH stroke scale is less than 4.
2. Stroke onset is clear and initiation of treatment can occur within 4.5 h. The earlier I.V. t-PA can be given even within the window, the better the outcome.
3. CT scan of the head shows *no* well-established acute infarct (more than 1/3 the MCA territory), no hemorrhage, brain tumor, or other etiology to explain the new focal neurological deficit.

Contraindications for I.V. t-PA:

1. Age less than 18 years.
2. CT scan of the head shows hemorrhage, tumor, abscess, well-established acute infarct (more than 1/3 the MCA territory), or arteriovenous malformation.
3. Rapidly resolving deficit, seizure, or suspected subarachnoid hemorrhage (absolute contraindication).
4. Stroke, significant head trauma, or intracranial surgery within the last 3 months (absolute contraindication).

5. History of intracranial hemorrhage, brain aneurysm, vascular malformation, or brain tumor.
6. Bacterial endocarditis.
7. Arterial puncture at a noncompressible site within 7 days.
8. Pregnancy or early postpartum (contraindication).
9. Liver or kidney biopsy, lumbar puncture, gastrointestinal, urological, or pulmonary hemorrhage within the last 3 weeks.
10. Known bleeding disorder or hemodialysis.
11. Platelets <100,000 (absolute contraindication).

   Current use of oral anticoagulant with INR >1.7 or PT >15 s *or* use of heparin within 48 h preceding stroke onset *and* prolonged aPTT at time of presentation
   Dabigatran use in the past 48 h (if last dose >48 h, confirm normal renal function [creatinine clearance >50 ml/min] and normal coagulation parameters [aPTT, INR, platelet count] before t-PA administration)
   Low molecular weight heparin use in the past 24 h

12. High blood pressure: systolic >185 mmHg or diastolic >110 mmHg, despite treatment to lower blood pressure acutely (absolute contraindication)
13. Significant hypo- [<50 mg/dl] or hyperglycemia [>400 mg/dl]. These are generally considered relative contraindications if deficits are quite severe (NIH stroke score >22 in 0–3 h *or* >25 in the 3–4.5-h window).

Administration of I.V. t-PA:

1. If criteria are met, start treatment within 4.5 h of onset (earliest within 3 h if possible).
2. The dose is 0.9 mg/kg to a maximum total dose of 90 mg. Ten percent of this dose is given as a bolus; the remainder is given over 60 min.
3. The patient should be closely monitored in the ICU for signs of hemorrhage and worsening neurological deficits.

4. Blood pressure must be well controlled (see below).
5. No adjunctive antiplatelet or anticoagulant medications are given for 24 h after I.V. thrombolysis.

Acute Antihypertensive Treatment After the Administration of t-PA [Target: 155–175/ 85–100 mmHg]

Monitor blood pressure (noninvasively) during the first 24 h after starting treatment as follows: every 15 min for 2 h, then every 30 min for 6 h, and then every 60 min until 24 h after starting treatment.

1. If systolic blood pressure is more than 180 mmHg or diastolic is more than 105 mmHg, on at least 2 readings 5–10 min apart, give:

   Labetalol 10 mg I.V. Repeat as needed every 10–20 min, doubling subsequent doses if necessary to a total cumulative dose of 70 mg, then consider labetalol drip. Monitor blood pressure every 15 min during labetalol treatment and observe closely for hypotension.

2. For hypertensive management with a heart rate of less than 60 per min, give hydralazine 5–20 mg I.V. q 20–30 min.
3. If there is no response to labetalol and/or hydralazine, administer nicardipine drip.

CT Scan Normal or Shows Ischemic Infarct and Patient Is Not a Candidate for t-PA

1. These patients should be assessed thoroughly with respect to the modifiable risk factors of stroke such as hypertension, diabetes mellitus, hypercholesterolemia, coronary artery

TABLE 18.1 The ABCD² score for stratifying subsequent stroke risk in transient ischemic attacks (TIAs)

ABCD² score for transient ischemic attacks (TIAs)					
Points	Age (years)	Blood pressure (mmHg)	Clinical features	Duration (min)	Diabetes
0	<60	Normal	Outside those specified	<10	No diabetes
1	≥60	Elevated (≥140/90)	Speech disturbance Without weakness	10–59	Has diabetes
2			Unilateral weakness	≥60	
Interpretation					
Low risk			Moderate risk	High risk	
0–3 points			4–5 points	6–7 points	
2-day stroke risk: 1.0 %			2-day stroke risk: 4.1 %	2-day stroke risk: 8.1 %	
7-day stroke risk: 1.2 %			7-day stroke risk: 5.9 %	7-day stroke risk: 11.7 %	
90-day stroke risk: 3.1 %			90-day stroke risk: 9.8 %	90-day stroke risk: 17.8 %	

disease, cardiac arrhythmias, carotid stenosis, and smoking. It is essential to modify the vascular risk factors to decrease the future risk of stroke and TIA.

Use the ABCD² score (Table 18.1) [4] to help triage TIA patients. Obtain ECG and carotid imaging within 24 h in all, and admit those with a score of more than or equal to four. Regardless of the score, all patients should eventually have a complete TIA/stroke work-up.

2. Start isotonic I.V. fluids such as normal saline.
3. Treat elevated temperature, manage hypo- and hyperglycemia, maintain good nutritional status, prevent deep vein thrombosis, minimize aspiration risks, and provide GI prophylaxis.
4. Start antiplatelet agents if no contraindications or allergies are known. If already on aspirin, determine if the stroke is due to *aspirin failure or failure to take aspirin*. Choose from the following:

   (a) Aspirin: loading dose 325 mg (optional); followed by 81 mg daily
   (b) Clopidogrel (Plavix®) 75 mg daily (the role of loading of clopidogrel in stroke is not well established)
   (c) Aggrenox® (dipyridamole 200/aspirin 25) twice a day

5. Check the fasting lipid profile. Start on cholesterol lowering agent such as atorvastatin or rosuvastatin. Target LDL ideally <70 mg/dl (1.8 mmol/l), especially if there are comorbid cardiovascular risk factors.
6. Avoid all antihypertensive medications for 24 h post-symptom onset. After this time, if there is a history of hypertension or diabetes mellitus, start/restart an ACE inhibitor such as ramipril, provided there are no contraindications.
7. If there is a history of cardiac arrhythmia such as atrial fibrillation, then anticoagulation with warfarin is indicated. Consider Holter monitor.
8. Do vascular imaging: carotid ultrasound and brain CT angiogram or MR angiogram.
9. If a cardiac embolic source is suspected and 2-D echocardiogram is negative, consider transesophageal echocardiogram (TEE).

Transient Ischemic Attack (TIA)

By traditional definition, symptoms of a TIA last less than 24 h, but usually symptoms resolve within 5–20 min. TIAs with speech and motor deficits are considered at higher risk for imminent stroke as compared to TIAs with minor sensory

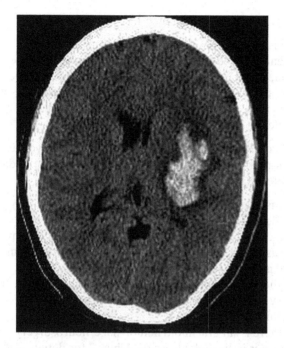

FIGURE 18.3 Non-contrasted head CT scan showing left intracerebral hemorrhage (Courtesy of Dr. R. Goh)

symptoms. *Stroke work-up should be done urgently in a high-risk (ABCD² score more than or equal to four) TIA patient to prevent stroke* (see section "CT Scan Normal or Shows Ischemic Infarct and Patient Is Not a Candidate for t-PA").

CT Scan Shows Hemorrhage (Hyperdensity)

Intracerebral hemorrhage (Fig. 18.3) may be primary or may be a secondary hemorrhagic conversion of an ischemic infarct.

1. Control of blood pressure is essential. Exact parameters are not well established and controversial. For patients with a MAP over 120 mmHg, a 10–15 % reduction in blood pressure is reasonable. However, reducing MAP below approximately 100 mmHg should be avoided.

Labetalol or nicardipine I.V. may be needed.

2. Start isotonic I.V. fluids such as normal saline.
3. Treat elevated temperature, manage hypo- and hyperglycemia, maintain good nutritional status, prevent deep vein thrombosis, provide GI prophylaxis, and minimize aspiration risks.
4. Rule out coagulopathy.

   Check PT, aPTT, INR, and platelet count. Give fresh frozen plasma 8 units every 4 h or vitamin K 10 mg daily or platelets if needed.

5. Consult neurosurgery.
6. Order MRI and MRA.
7. If ischemic infarct with secondary hemorrhagic conversion is suspected, cardiac monitoring, 2-D echocardiogram, and a full ischemic stroke work-up are indicated.
8. If there is an epidural or subdural hemorrhage, neurosurgery consultation is indicated. Please see Chap. 8 for details.
9. If there is subarachnoid hemorrhage, neurosurgery consultation is indicated. Please see Chap. 7 for details.

Discussion

Complications

1. Herniation (Fig. 18.4)
   Uncal herniation is seen in large strokes. The patient becomes more lethargic with progressive deterioration of the mental status. The pupil may be dilated and fixed or sluggish to light. A stat CT scan is indicated if the herniation is suspected. The patient also requires intubation and hyperventilation. Mannitol 1 g/kg titrated to serum osmolality is started. Neurosurgical consultation for possible hemicraniectomy is required [5]. Hypotonic fluids are avoided; hypertonic saline may be utilized with close monitoring of serum sodium and osmolality.

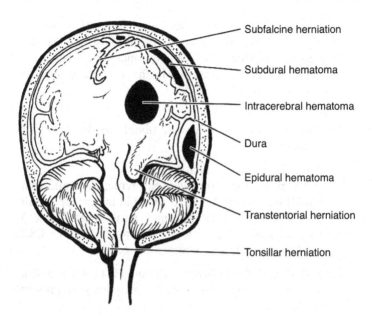

- Subfalcine herniation
- Subdural hematoma
- Intracerebral hematoma
- Dura
- Epidural hematoma
- Transtentorial herniation
- Tonsillar herniation

FIGURE 18.4 Herniation syndromes and major focal intracranial hemorrhage types

2. Hemorrhagic Conversion

Hemorrhagic conversion of ischemic stroke may be asymptomatic or characterized by sudden clinical deterioration. This is seen mostly in large embolic strokes. Antiplatelet and anticoagulant therapy is generally stopped for at least 3–4 weeks, and neurosurgical consultation is obtained.

3. Recurrent Strokes

Recurrent stroke within 30 days may occur in about 5 % of patients, especially those who have carotid stenosis or cardioembolic disease.

4. Extension of Current Ischemic Territory

Extension of current ischemic territory due to progressive thrombosis, more proximal occlusion of carotid circulation, or aggressive lowering of blood pressure is not uncommon. The precipitating factors are avoided, adequate volume status is maintained, and blood pressure should not be lowered aggressively. Heparin may be helpful in these patients. The preventative treatment for recurrent stroke includes aggressive management of the above-mentioned risk factors and carotid endarterectomy if the carotid stenosis is significant (generally if >70 %).

5. Stroke in a Young Patient
   Young patients require additional stroke work-up, including:

   1. A thrombophilia evaluation:
      serum protein C and protein S; a screen for antithrombin III deficiency; ANA, rheumatoid factor; lupus anticoagulant and anticardiolipin antibodies; factor V Leiden/activated protein C resistance; VDRL; ESR; C3, C4, and CH50; and homocysteine.

   2. MRA and MR venogram and beta HCG if any indication of venous thrombosis or pregnancy is present/suspected.

   3. Transesophageal echocardiogram (TEE).

References

1. Easton JD, Saver JL, Albers GW, Alberts MJ, Chaturvedi S, Feldmann E, Hatsukami TS, Higashida RT, Johnston SC, Kidwell CS, Lutsep HL, Miller E, Sacco RL. Definition and evaluation of transient ischemic attack: a scientific statement for healthcare professionals from the American Heart Association/American Stroke Association Stroke Council; Council on Cardiovascular Surgery and Anesthesia; Council on Cardiovascular Radiology and Intervention; Council on Cardiovascular Nursing; and the Interdisciplinary Council on Peripheral Vascular Disease. Stroke. 2009;40(6):2276–93.
2. Messé SR, Fonarow GC, Smith EE, Kaltenbach L, Olson DM, Kasner SE, Schwamm LH. Use of tissue-type plasminogen activator before and after publication of the European Cooperative Acute Stroke Study III in Get With The Guidelines-Stroke. Circ Cardiovasc Qual Outcomes. 2012;5(3):321–6.
3. Merino JG, Warach S. Imaging of acute stroke. Nat Rev Neurol. 2010;6(10):560–71.

4. Rothwell PM, Giles MF, Flossmann E, Lovelock CE, Redgrave JN, Warlow CP, Mehta Z. A simple score (ABCD) to identify individuals at high early risk of stroke after transient ischaemic attack. Lancet. 2005;366(9479):29–36.
5. Arnaout OM, Aoun SG, Batjer HH, Bendok BR. Decompressive hemicraniectomy after malignant middle cerebral artery infarction: rationale and controversies. Neurosurg Focus. 2011; 30(6):E18.

Chapter 19
Syncope

1. *Syncope* is a brief loss of consciousness due to sudden, global transient reduction in blood supply to the brain.
2. *Presyncope* is due to similar causes as syncope; however, patients have transitory altered but not complete loss of consciousness.

Characteristic features include:

1. Loss of consciousness (syncope) lasting anywhere from a few seconds to a few minutes
2. No aura or postictal confusion
3. Feelings of generalized weakness, lightheadedness, or dizziness
4. Profuse diaphoresis, palpitations, and pallor with cold extremities
5. Minor twitching or trembling and even convulsions (convulsive syncope)
6. Rarely urinary incontinence

The most important task is to rule out serious causes such as cardiac arrhythmias, myocardial ischemia/infarction, pulmonary embolism, GI bleed with shock, carotid or aortic dissection, intracranial bleeding, and seizures.

Stabilize the Patient

ABCs

1. Assess the airway and breathing rate, and look for signs of respiratory distress.

A.Q. Rana, J.A. Morren, *Neurological Emergencies in Clinical Practice,* DOI 10.1007/978-1-4471-5191-3_19, © Springer-Verlag London 2013

2. Check the vital signs and assess if the patient is hemodynamically stable. Place the patient on a cardiac monitor and pulse oximeter. Patients may have hypotension (possibly orthostatic) or bradycardia. Start I.V. fluids if needed.

Focused History

Take a focused history of the presenting symptom and the onset.

Focused Exam

Do a focused neurological exam. Assess the current level of consciousness. Most patients regain consciousness very quickly by the time the neurology service is called. If the patient is still unconscious, then turn the patient to the left lateral decubitus position and manage as a comatose patient (see Chap. 1).

STAT Labs and Treatments

1. Check the finger-stick glucose. Give thiamine 100 mg I.V., then 50 ml of D50W intravenously if indicated.
2. Obtain ECG with rhythm strip.

Identify the Underlying Cause

Take Further History

1. Ask if the patient actually did lose consciousness.
2. Ask about the circumstances when the patient lost consciousness. Were they lying, sitting, or standing at the onset? Syncope in the supine position is almost always due to cardiac causes, whereas syncope immediately after standing up suggests orthostatic hypotension.

3. Ask if there was there any seizure-like activity, tongue biting, or incontinence of bowel or bladder. Find out if the episode was preceded by an aura and if it was followed by slow sensorium recovery.
4. Ask if there was any head injury, sudden severe headache, or neck pain.
5. Ask if this was the first episode and if the patient had any warnings, dimming of vision, lightheadedness, pallor, or diaphoresis which are usually due to reflex vasodepressor syncope.
6. Ask if the syncope occurred after turning the head suddenly to one side, such as in carotid sinus syncope.
7. Ask if the syncope was preceded by Valsalva maneuver such as in micturition, defecation, or cough.
8. Ask about diplopia, dysarthria, dysphagia, vertigo, numbness, weakness, and bowel and bladder symptoms which could be seen in vertebrobasilar insufficiency or brainstem TIA. *A TIA involving the brain stem can cause a brief decline in the level of consciousness.*

Do Further Examination

1. A complete neurological examination should be done. This includes testing mental status, cranial nerves, muscle bulk, tone, power, adventitious movements, deep tendon reflexes, plantar responses, coordination with station and gait assessment, as well as sensory examination of all modalities.
2. Cranial nerve examination. Check for:

    (a) *Papilledema* which can occur in mass lesions causing increased intracranial pressure
    (b) *Subhyaloid hemorrhages* which occur in subarachnoid hemorrhage
    (c) *Hemianopsia* seen in stroke and mass lesions

3. Motor and sensory examination. Check for:

    (a) *Pronator drift, focal weakness, hemisensory loss, incoordination or binocular visual deficits* which are seen in mass lesions, intracranial bleeding, or stroke

(b) *Sensory loss in glove and stocking distribution* which is seen in peripheral neuropathy potentially having an autonomic component as well

(c) *Tremor, rigidity, bradykinesia*, and other signs of Parkinsonism

4. Look for meningeal signs.

Brudzinski's sign is present if passive flexion of the patient's neck by the examiner results in flexion of the lower extremities.

Kernig's sign is present if, with hip and knee in flexion, passive extension of the knee is restricted by hamstring spasm and/or pain.

Meningeal signs have low sensitivity and specificity. Neck stiffness with extension and flexion but normal rotation is a more reliable sign of meningitis. Also, meningismus is not specific to infection but can be seen in subarachnoid hemorrhage.

5. Inspect the tongue for laceration.

6. Inspect for signs of trauma.

Those which indicate a fracture at the base of the skull include:

Battle's sign: ecchymosis over the mastoid process

Raccoon eyes: ecchymosis around the periorbital area

There may also be CSF rhinorrhea or CSF otorrhea present.

7. Check blood pressure in both supine and erect position. Assess for an orthostatic change (>20 mmHg in systolic and/or >10 mmHg in diastolic pressures).

8. Examine cardiovascular, respiratory, and GI systems. Keep aortic dissection and GI bleed in mind.

Do Further Investigations

1. Send blood work: CBC and CMP (especially electrolytes and blood glucose).

2. If neurological causes are suspected, order:

(a) CT/MRI brain scan

(b) EEG to rule out seizure activity

(c) Carotid ultrasound, cardiac monitoring, and 2-D echocardiogram

3. If subarachnoid hemorrhage is suspected and CT is negative, patients need a lumbar puncture.

    All syncope patients require electrocardiography (including QT interval monitoring) and orthostatic vital signs. Patients with established cardiovascular disease, abnormality on electrocardiography, or a family history of sudden death and those with unexplained syncope require admission for further diagnostic evaluation [1].

Treat the Underlying Cause

Treatment depends on the underlying cause and frequently requires a cardiology referral. True neurological causes of syncope are found only in about 5–10 % of cases. The majority of cases are due to reflex vasodilatation, transient drop in blood pressure, cardiac arrhythmias, or orthostatic hypotension.

1. Reflex Vasodilatation (Vasodepressor Response)

    This is the most common cause of a syncopal episode. The etiology may be vasovagal, neurocardiogenic, carotid sinus syncope, postmicturition, postdefecation, or cough-induced syncope. It can also be associated with pain.

2. Postural Hypotension

    This may result from dehydration/hypovolemia, anemia, or medications.

3. Cardiac Causes

    This is the second most common cause of syncopal episodes and includes sick sinus syndrome, second and third degree AV block, supraventricular and ventricular tachycardia, ventricular fibrillation, pacemaker malfunction, aortic and mitral valve stenosis and hypertrophic obstructive cardiomyopathy. Vascular etiologies include subclavian steal syndrome.

4. Neurological Causes

    These account for a minority of syncopal episodes. Patients may have orthostatic hypotension from autonomic dysfunction such as that seen in Parkinson's disease and multiple system atrophy (especially in Shy-Drager syndrome). Bilateral carotid stenosis, vertebrobasilar stenosis, brainstem

TIA, seizure, focal mass lesions, intracranial hemorrhage including subarachnoid hemorrhage may present with syncope, but other clinical features usually predominate.

5. Other Causes

Psychiatric and miscellaneous causes such as emotional stress, hyperventilation, and prolonged extension of the neck in patients with extracranial atherosclerotic disease can cause syncope.

Discussion

Twitching and even convulsions can be seen in syncope and is not necessarily indicative of a seizure [2]. Incontinence is usually an indicator of seizure but can also be seen in syncope.

Medications Commonly Causing Syncope

1. Calcium channel blockers
2. ACE inhibitors
3. Beta-blockers
4. Diuretics
5. Antiarrhythmic agents such as procainamide, quinidine, sotalol, and amiodarone
6. Monoamine oxidase inhibitors
7. Tricyclic antidepressants
8. Dopamine agonists and levodopa
9. Digoxin

References

1. Gauer RL. Evaluation of syncope. Am Fam Physician. 2011;84(6):640–50.
2. Hart YM. All that shakes is not epilepsy. J R Coll Physicians Edinb. 2012;42(2):151–4.

Chapter 20
Transient Global Amnesia (TGA)

Patients with transient global amnesia (TGA) are typically middle-aged or elderly who are usually brought to the emergency department by a relative describing the patient as being "confused." There are no focal neurological deficits, and cognitive as well as language functions are intact. However, there is a profound anterograde more than retrograde amnesia for the preceding several hours or a day. Patients are usually quite agitated and may repeat the same question (previously answered) over and over, such as "What am I doing here? Where am I?" Over time, the anterograde amnesia subsides and usually resolves completely. TGA may often appear in the setting of an emotional or physical stress [1].

Stabilize the Patient

ABCs

1. Assess the airway and breathing rate, and look for signs of respiratory distress. Check the vital signs and assess if the patient is hemodynamically stable. Place the patient on a cardiac monitor and pulse oximeter. Most patients are stable.
2. Use a quiet room if possible. Provide reorientation and reassurance to the patient.

A.Q. Rana, J.A. Morren, *Neurological Emergencies in Clinical Practice,* DOI 10.1007/978-1-4471-5191-3_20, © Springer-Verlag London 2013

Focused History

1. Ask about the presenting symptoms, time of onset, and if progressive or not. These can include questions such as "What is the last thing you remember?"
2. Ask questions to rule out any other causes of the presenting symptoms, such as a transient ischemic attack, a seizure, or head trauma.

Focused Exam

1. Check for orientation, naming, repetition, fluency, comprehension, visual fields, facial and limb weakness, pronator drift, coordination and plantar responses.

Initial Labs

Finger-stick glucose, CBC, CMP, and ECG +/- toxicology screen.

Identify the Underlying Cause

Take Further History

1. Ask about any additional symptoms, such as speech problems, anxiety, depression, numbness, and weakness.
2. Ask about any stressful events, physical or emotional, that may have occurred leading up to the attack. Patients may mention strong physical exertion prior to the event or some type of emotional stress that is not disclosed initially.
3. Ask about the onset of memory loss. Was it sudden onset or gradual? How long it lasted? Any other precipitating events? Any aura? Did patient look bewildered to the others? Or were they repeating the same thing again and again? Is memory loss now improving or not? Find out if there were any previous similar episodes.

4. Ask about the recent use of pertinent medications, especially benzodiazepines which can commonly cause episodic amnesia.

Do Further Examination

A complete neurological examination should be done. This includes testing mental status, cranial nerves, muscle bulk, tone, power, adventitious movements, deep tendon reflexes, plantar responses, coordination with station and gait assessment, as well as sensory examination of all modalities.

Do Further Investigations

1. Investigations may be required to rule out other possible causes of the amnesia. Exclusion of other neurological conditions such as stroke, seizure, or migraine episodes which can present with a similar type of memory disturbance is important.
2. Electroencephalogram (EEG) can help to assess for any interictal epileptic discharges in cases of epilepsy.
3. Head CT scan or MRI is useful in determining mass lesions or possible vascular causes such as stroke.

Treat the Underlying Cause

The exact pathophysiology of transient global amnesia still remains unclear. As such, both epileptic and vascular mechanisms have been proposed but have not been proven. The condition is self-limiting and there is no specific treatment.

Discussion

The prognosis of TGA is usually good. The rate of recurrence is low, generally occurring in about 8 % of patients [2].

The attacks of amnesia should have been observed by a witness and reported as having a definitive loss of short-term memory. No focal deficits, cognitive impairment, loss of consciousness, history of seizures or epilepsy, or head trauma should be present which may suggest a secondary cause for the amnesia. The attack typically subsides within 24 h with a gradual return of memory. Patients do not have the capability to create new memories of events during the episodes, but otherwise they are mentally attentive, stable, and alert. They retain full memory of self-identity and that of close contacts. They also maintain perceptual skills along with complex learned behaviors. The attack may be accompanied with anxiety, and a common symptom is repetitive questioning: usually questions which were answered satisfactorily earlier during the episode.

References

1. Hunter G. Transient global amnesia. Neurol Clin. 2011;29(4): 1045–54.
2. Pantoni L, Bertini E, Lamassa M, Pracucci G, Inzitari D. Clinical features, risk factors and prognosis in transient global amnesia: a follow-up study. Eur J Neurol. 2005;12:350–6.

Chapter 21
Visual Impairments

Most patients referred to the neurology service for visual disturbances have a chief complaint of blurred vision, double vision, or acute loss of vision. The visual symptoms may be either a positive or a negative phenomenon.

Positive phenomena: Light flashes, bright spots, scintillating scotomas, photopsia, phosphenes, and zigzag lines starting small and enlarging with fortifications (fortification spectra). These are usually seen in patients with migraine or epilepsy.

Negative phenomena: Blindness, visual field deficits or scotomas, decreased visual acuity, and color blindness or desaturation. These are usually seen in conditions like stroke, multiple sclerosis and neuromyelitis optica.

Stabilize the Patient

ABCs

1. Assess the airway and breathing rate, and look for signs of respiratory distress.
2. Check the vital signs and assess if the patient is hemodynamically stable. Place the patient on a cardiac monitor and pulse oximeter. Most patients will be stable.

A.Q. Rana, J.A. Morren, *Neurological Emergencies in Clinical Practice,* DOI 10.1007/978-1-4471-5191-3_21, © Springer-Verlag London 2013

Focused History

1. Take a focused history of the presenting symptom including onset and temporal evolution.
2. Ask about acute trauma.

Identify the Underlying Cause

Take Further History

1. Ask if the visual symptom involves one or both eyes.

   One eye (*monocular*): localizes to the eye, retina, or optic nerve

   Both eyes (*binocular*): localizes to the optic chiasm or along the pathway to the occipital lobes (retrochiasmal lesions)

2. Ask the exact nature of the symptoms.
   Specify whether the chief complaint is blurred vision, double vision, loss of vision, light flashes, zigzag lines, or transient visual obscurations.

   Blurred vision or loss of vision: usually ischemic and may be from optic neuritis (which can be ischemic, demyelinating, or inflammatory)

   Double vision: seen in neuromuscular diseases such as myasthenia gravis and cranial nerves III, IV, and VI palsy from any cause

   Transient visual obscurations (*dimming of vision lasting seconds*): often occur with change in position and are seen in pseudotumor cerebri

3. Ask about the onset.

   Onset over seconds to minutes: usually vascular

   Onset over hours: anterior ischemic optic neuropathy or pseudotumor cerebri

   Onset over days: retrobulbar lesions- demyelinating lesion and neoplasm

4. If the patient complains of double vision, ask if it disappears on closing one eye. If diplopia is monocular, the cause is usually ocular, such as lens/refractory or retinal pathology or factitious/functional.

5. For diplopia: Ask if the two images are horizontal, diagonal, or vertical.

> *Horizontal*: cranial nerves III and VI involvement
> *Vertical and diagonal*: cranial nerve IV (and possible cranial nerve III) involvement

6. Ask about symptoms and risk factors associated with diplopia:

> *Ptosis, fluctuating weakness, and speech and swallowing problems*: suggest myasthenia gravis
> *Vascular risk factors*: favor cranial nerve palsies due to ischemia or aneurysm
> *Headaches, fever, chills, weight loss, jaw and tongue claudication, and myalgias*: suggest temporal arteritis (arteritic anterior ischemic optic neuropathy), especially in elderly patients [1, 2]
> *Eye pain*: suggests optic neuritis.
> *Weakness, sensory symptoms, bladder and bowel problems, Lhermitte's symptom, and Uhthoff's phenomenon*: suggest multiple sclerosis.

Do Examination

A complete neurological examination should be done. This includes testing mental status, cranial nerves, muscle bulk, tone, power, adventitious movements, deep tendon reflexes, plantar responses, coordination with station and gait assessment, as well as sensory examination of all modalities.

1. Mental status.

   (a) Assess for dysarthria that could be seen with jaw and tongue claudication.

2. Cranial nerve examination.

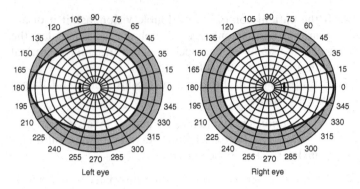

FIGURE 21.1 Normal visual fields

(a) Do fundoscopy for changes related to papilledema, optic neuritis, and optic atrophy as well as retinal artery or vein occlusion.

(b) Check visual fields to confrontation. Normal visual fields on formal testing are illustrated in Fig. 21.1.

> *Unilateral visual loss*: prechiasmatic-retinal or optic nerve involvement (Fig. 21.2)
>
> *Hemianopsia*: lesion of visual pathway from optic chiasm to occipital lobe (Fig. 21.3)
>
> *Superior quadrantanopia* (*"pie in the sky" pattern of deficit*): inferior optic radiation involvement due to a temporal lobe lesion (Fig. 21.4)
>
> *Inferior quadrantanopia* (*"pie on the floor" pattern of deficit*): superior optic radiation involvement in a parietal lobe lesion (Fig. 21.5)

(c) Check visual acuity with hand-held Snellen chart (with best possible correction).

(d) Check color vision using Ishihara color plates. Also look for red desaturation.

(e) Examine pupillary size, shape, regularity, reactivity to light and accommodation and relative afferent pupillary defect (RAPD).

(f) Look for gaze deviation.

> *Away from hemiparesis*: (destructive) cortical lesion

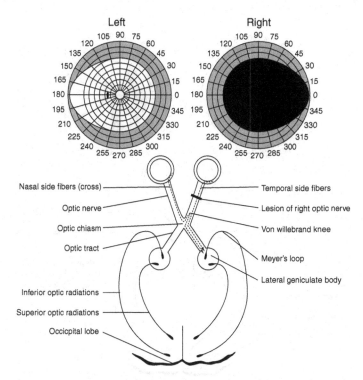

FIGURE 21.2 Right-sided visual field defect due to complete right optic nerve lesion

> *Toward the hemiparesis*: pontine lesion (Millard-Gubler syndrome)

(g) Examine extraocular movements. Note the position of the eye in primary position first. Check eye movements in all directions.

> *Eye down and out in primary position*: cranial nerve III involvement (Fig. 1.1)
>
> *Internuclear ophthalmoplegia (INO)*: brainstem lesions involving ipsilateral medial longitudinal fasciculus (MLF). There is impaired adduction of the ipsilateral eye and abduction nystagmus of the contralateral eye (Fig. 21.6).

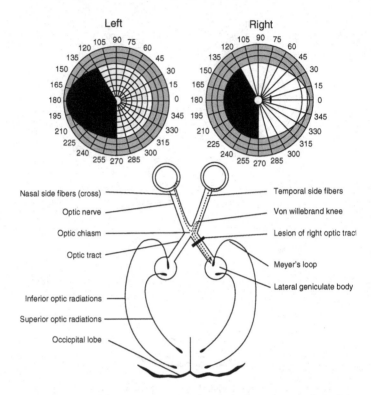

FIGURE 21.3 Left homonymous hemianopsia due to a complete right optic tract lesion

> *One and a half syndrome*: ipsilateral paramedian pontine reticular formation (PPRF) or cranial nerve VI nuclear lesion with ipsilateral MLF lesion. The only horizontal eye movement possible is abduction of the contralateral eye. Convergence is usually spared [3].

3. Motor and sensory examination.

   (a) Assess for hemineglect/inattention which may mimic a cortical visual deficit. Also check for hemiparesis (as can be seen in Millard-Gubler syndrome).

4. Palpate temporal arteries for tenderness (seen in temporal arteritis).

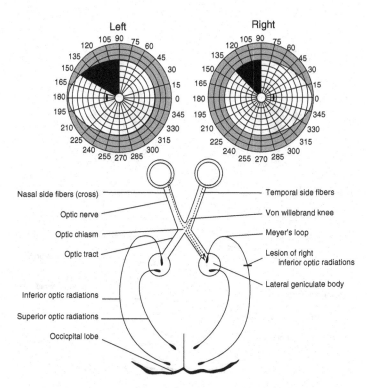

FIGURE 21.4 Left superior quadrantanopia ("pie in the sky" defect) due to lesion of right inferior optic radiations (or Meyer's loop)

Do Investigations

Investigations depend on the suspected cause but *may* include:

1. Blood work: CBC, ESR, CRP, TSH, PT, INR, fasting lipid profile, serum glucose, and HbA1c.
2. Brain (+/− orbit-dedicated) MRI and brain MRA, carotid ultrasound, and 2-D echocardiogram.
3. EEG.
4. If optic neuritis is suspected, may order visual evoked potential (VEP) study

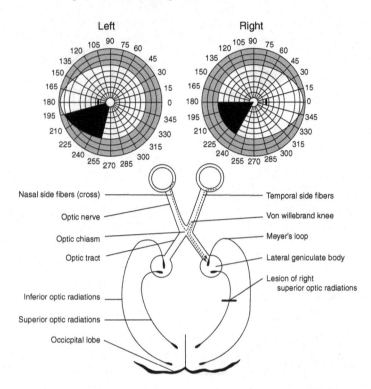

FIGURE 21.5 Left inferior quadrantanopia due to lesion of right superior optic radiations

5. If myasthenia gravis is suspected, acetylcholine receptor and MuSK antibodies, repetitive nerve stimulation testing (+/− single-fiber EMG), and CT scan of the chest.
6. Neuro-ophthalmology referral.

Treat the Underlying Cause

Treatment depends on the underlying cause (see section "Discussion").

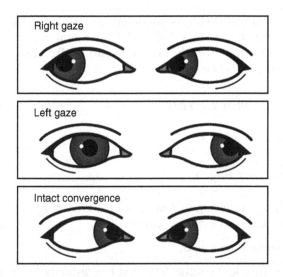

FIGURE 21.6 Internuclear ophthalmoplegia (INO) of the right side-impaired adduction of the right eye and abduction nystagmus of the left eye upon left horizontal gaze

Discussion

Anterior Ischemic Optic Neuropathy

Please see Chap. 5.

Demyelinating Optic Neuritis

This usually occurs in young patients, more female than male when multiple sclerosis is causal. However, Devic's disease (neuromyelitis optica) is a diagnostic possibility.

> *Investigations*: Contrasted MRI of the brain and orbits and Visual evoked potentials are abnormal. Aquaporin-4-specific serum autoantibody may be positive in neuromyelitis optica.

Treatment: Methylprednisolone (Solu-Medrol®) 1 g I.V. daily for 3 days followed by an oral steroid taper (according to the Optic Neuritis Treatment Trial (ONTT)) [4–6].

Pseudotumor Cerebri

Please see Chap. 15.

Amaurosis Fugax

This may be the equivalent of a TIA, indicating high-grade carotid stenosis or embolic disease.

Symptoms and signs:

(a) Transient monocular vision loss lasting a few minutes to half an hour.
(b) Described as a shade or a curtain coming down over the eye (respects the horizontal meridian).
(c) There is no pain.
(d) May have stroke risk factors (hypertension, diabetes mellitus, dyslipidemia, smoking, coronary artery disease, hypercoagulable disorder or cardiac arrhythmias).

Investigations
Full stroke workup including brain neuroimaging and carotid Doppler or MRA and 2-D echocardiogram +/– Holter monitor
Treatment:

(a) Antiplatelet agents
(b) If >70 % stenosis of the ipsilateral carotid artery, carotid endarterectomy is generally recommended.

Retinal Vessel Occlusion

This is usually apparent on retinal examination. Ophthalmology consultation is required.

References

1. Hayreh SS. Anterior ischemic optic neuropathy. Clin Neurosci. 1997;4(5):251–63.
2. Unwin B, Williams CM, Gilliland W. Polymyalgia rheumatica and giant cell arteritis. Am Fam Physician. 2006;74(9):1547–54.
3. Glaser JS. Neuro-ophthalmology. 3rd ed. Philadelphia: Lippincott Williams & Wilkins; 1999.
4. Beck RW, Cleary PA, Trobe JD, et al. The effect of corticosteroids for acute optic neuritis on the subsequent development of multiple sclerosis. N Engl J Med. 1993;329:1764–9.
5. Beck RW, Cleary PA, Optic Neuritis Study Group. Optic neuritis treatment trial: one-year follow-up results. Arch Ophthalmol. 1993;111:773–5.
6. Beck RW, Cleary PA. The optic neuritis treatment trial: three-year follow-up results. Arch Ophthalmol. 1995;113:136.

Appendices

Appendix 1: Nerves and Root Supply of Muscles

Upper limb	Spinal roots
Spinal accessory nerve	
Trapezius	C3, C4
Brachial plexus	
Rhomboids – dorsal scapular nerve	C5
Serratus anterior – long thoracic nerve	C5, C6, C7
Pectoralis major	
Clavicular ⎱	C5, C6, C7
Sternal ⎰	C8, T1
Supraspinatus	**C5**, C6
Infraspinatus	C5, C6
Latissimus dorsi – thoracodorsal nerve	C6, C7, C8
Teres major – subscapular nerve	C5, C6, C7
Axillary nerve	
Deltoid	**C5**, C6
Musculocutaneous nerve	
Biceps	C5, C6

(continued)

A.Q. Rana, J.A. Morren, *Neurological Emergencies in Clinical Practice,* DOI 10.1007/978-1-4471-5191-3, © Springer-Verlag London 2013

Appendix 1   (continued)

Upper limb	Spinal roots
Brachialis	C5, C6
Radial nerve	
Triceps: long, lateral and medial head	C6, **C7**, C8
Brachioradialis	C5, C6
Extensor carpi radialis longus – wrist extension	C6, C7
Posterior interosseous nerve	
Supinator	C6, C7
Extensor carpi ulnaris	C7, C8
Extensor digitorum	C7, C8
Abductor pollicis longus	C7, C8
Extensor pollicis longus	C7, C8
Extensor pollicis brevis	C7, **C8**
Extensor indicis	C7, **C8**
Extensor digiti minimi	C7, C8
Median nerve	
Pronator teres	C6, C7
Flexor carpi radialis	C6, C7
Flexor digitorum superficialis	C7, C8, T1
Abductor pollicis brevis	C8, T1
Flexor pollicis brevis[a] (usually superficial head)	C8, T1
Opponens pollicis	C8, T1
Lumbricals I and II	C8, T1
Anterior interosseous nerve	
Pronator quadratus	C7, C8
Flexor digitorum profundus I and II	C8, T1
Flexor pollicis longus	*C8*, T1

(continued)

Upper limb	Spinal roots
Ulnar nerve	
Flexor carpi ulnaris	C7, **C8**, T1
Flexor digitorum profundus III and IV	C8, T1
Abductor digiti minimi (hypothenar muscle)	C8, T1
Adductor pollicis	C8, T1
Flexor pollicis brevis[a] (usually deep head)	C8, T1
Palmar interossei	C8, T1
Dorsal interossei	C8, T1
Lumbricals III and IV	C8, T1

Lower limb	Spinal roots
Femoral nerve	
Iliopsoas	L1, L2, L3
Rectus femoris	L2, **L3**, **L4**
Vastus lateralis	
Vastus intermedius	
Vastus medialis	
Obturator nerve	
Adductor longus	L2, **L3**, **L4**
Adductor magnus[b] (adductor part)	
Superior gluteal nerve	
Gluteus medius and minimus	L4, **L5**, S1
Tensor fasciae latae	
Inferior gluteal nerve	
Gluteus maximus	L5, **S1**, S2
Sciatic and tibial nerve	
Semitendinosus	**L5**, S1, S2
Biceps femoris	**S1**, S2
Semimembranosus	**L5**, S1

(continued)

Appendix 1   (continued)

Lower limb	Spinal roots
Adductor magnus[b] (hamstring/ischiocondylar part)	L4
Gastrocnemius and soleus	**S1**, S2
Tibialis posterior	**L5**, S1
Flexor digitorum longus	**L5**, S1
Abductor hallucis Abductor digiti minimi Interossei of the foot	S1, S2
Sciatic and common peroneal nerve	
Tibialis anterior	L4, **L5**
Extensor digitorum longus	L5, S1
Extensor hallucis longus	L5
Extensor digitorum brevis	L5, S1
Peroneus longus	**L5**, S1
Peroneus brevis	L5, S1

This list includes only commonly tested muscles and does not include all the muscles innervated by the respective nerves

[a]The flexor pollicis brevis is usually dually supplied by the median and ulnar nerves

[b]Adductor magnus is dually supplied by the obturator nerve (adductor portion) and the tibial division of the sciatic nerve (hamstring/ischiocondylar portion)

Appendix 2: Commonly Tested Movements

Movement	Weakness (UMN)	Root	Reflex	Nerve	Muscle
Upper limb					
Shoulder abduction	++	C5/6		Axillary	Deltoid
Elbow flexion		C5/6	+	Musculocutaneous	Biceps
		C5/6	+	Radial	Brachioradialis
Elbow extension	+	C7	+	Radial	Triceps
Radial wrist extension	+	C6/7		Radial	Extensor carpi radialis longus
Finger extension	+	C7		Posterior interosseous nerve	Extensor digitorum communis
Finger flexion		C8/T1	+	Anterior interosseous nerve	Flexor pollicis longus + flexor digitorum profundus (digits 2 and 3)
				Ulnar	Flexor digitorum profundus (digits 4 and 5)

(continued)

Appendix 2   (continued)

Movement	Weakness (UMN)	Root	Reflex	Nerve	Muscle
Finger abduction	++	C8/T1		Ulnar	First dorsal interosseous
		C8/T1		Median	Abductor pollicis brevis
Lower limb					
Hip flexion	++	L1/2/3		Direct L1/2 branches, femoral	Iliopsoas
Hip adduction		L2/3/4	+	Obturator	Adductors
Hip extension		L5/S1		Inferior gluteal nerve	Gluteus maximus
Knee flexion	+	L5/S1		Sciatic	Hamstring
Knee extension		L3/4	+	Femoral	Quadriceps
Foot dorsiflexion	++	L4/5		Deep peroneal	Tibialis anterior
Foot eversion		L5/S1		Superficial peroneal	Peronei
Foot inversion		L5/S1		Tibial	Tibialis posterior
Plantar flexion		S1/S2	+	Tibial	Gastrocnemius, soleus

Appendix 3: Sensory Dermatomes

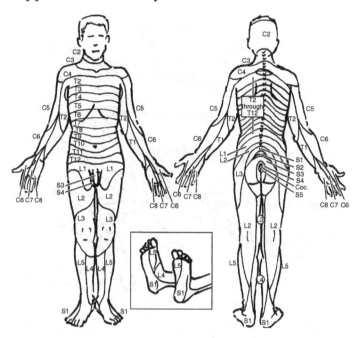

Appendix 4: Brachial Plexus

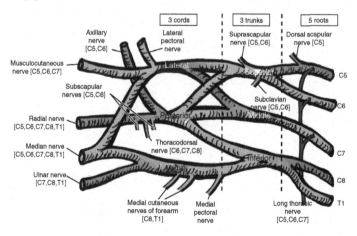

Appendix 5: Lumbar Plexus

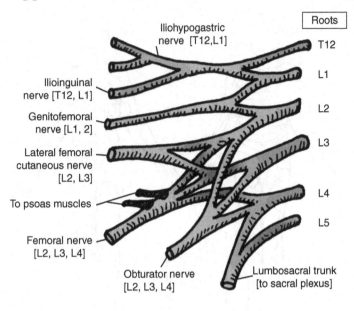

Roots

Iliohypogastric
nerve [T12,L1]

Ilioinguinal
nerve [T12, L1]

Genitofemoral
nerve [L1, 2]

Lateral femoral
cutaneous nerve
[L2, L3]

To psoas muscles

Femoral nerve
[L2, L3, L4]

Obturator nerve
[L2, L3, L4]

Lumbosacral trunk
[to sacral plexus]

T12

L1

L2

L3

L4

L5

Appendix 6: Muscles Supplied by Various Nerves

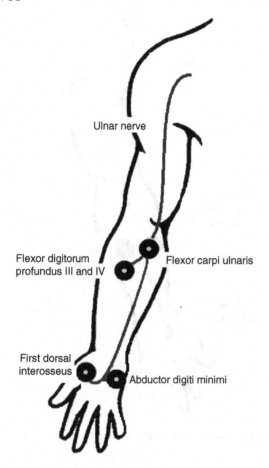

Muscles supplied by the ulnar nerve

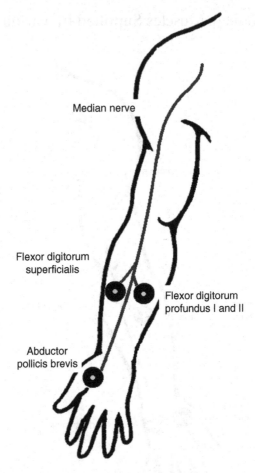

Muscles supplied by the median nerve

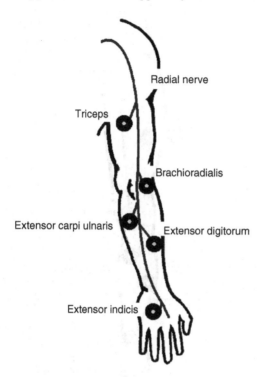

Muscles supplied by the radial nerve

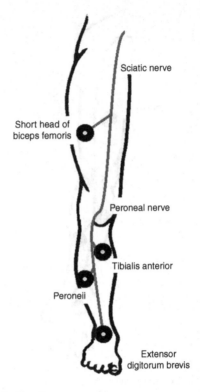

Muscles supplied by the peroneal nerve

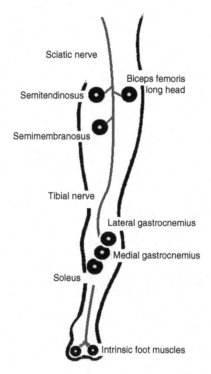

Muscles supplied by the tibial nerve

Index

A.Q. Rana, J.A. Morren, *Neurological Emergencies*
in Clinical Practice, DOI 10.1007/978-1-4471-5191-3,
© Springer-Verlag London 2013